to Chronic
Wound Repair

Contributors

Richard M. Allman, MD
Division of Gerontology and Geriatric Medicine
University of Alabama at Birmingham and
Birmingham Veterans Affairs Medical Center
Birmingham, AL

Patricia S. Goode, RN, ET, MSN, MD
Division of Gerontology and Geriatric Medicine
University of Alabama at Birmingham
Birmingham, AL

Patricia A. Haberer, MA, BSN, RN, CETN
Clinical Education Manager
Smith & Nephew, Inc.
Palm Harbor, FL

Katherine F. Jeter, ET, EdD
Spartanburg, SC

Karen Lou Kennedy, RN, CS, FNP
Family Nurse Practitioner, Skin and Wound Care
Fort Wayne, IN

William C. Krupski, MD
Professor of Surgery, Vascular Surgery Section
University of Colorado Health Sciences Center
Denver, CO

Gerit D. Mulder, DPM, MS
Director, Education & Research
University of California San Diego
San Diego, CA

Wayne J. Schroeder, MD
Senior Medical Director
Kinetic Concepts, Inc.
San Antonio, TX

Joseph B. Warren, BSN, RN, ET, CNRN
Program Director, Nursing Research Service
Brooke Army Medical Center
Fort Sam Houston, TX

Clinicians' Pocket Guide to Chronic Wound Repair

Fourth Edition

Editors
Gerit D. Mulder, DPM, MS
Patricia A. Haberer, MA, BSN, RN, CETN
Katherine F. Jeter, ET, EdD

WCCN
Wound Care Communications Network
Springhouse Corporation
Springhouse, PA

Printed in the United States of America.

CPGCWR-041098

ℝ A member of the Reed Elsevier plc group

Library of Congress Cataloging-in-Publication Data

Clinicians' pocket guide to chronic wound repair/editors, Gerit D. Mulder, Patricia A. Haberer, Katherine F. Jeter.--4th ed. p. cm.
Includes bibliographical references.
1. Wound healing--Handbooks, manuals, etc. 2. Wounds and injuries--Treatment--Handbooks, manuals, etc. I. Mulder, Gerit D. II. Haberer, Patricia A. III. Jeter, Katherine F. [DNLM: 1. Wounds and Injuries--therapy handbooks. 2. Wound Healing handbooks. 3. Skin Ulcer--therapy handbooks. WO 39 C64 1999]
RD94.C56   1998
617.1'406--dc21
DNLM/DLC   98-29793
ISBN 0-87434-988-5   CIP

Contents

Illustrations

Tables

Introduction

The Wound Healing Society defines *chronic wounds* as wounds that "fail to progress through a normal, orderly and timely sequence of repair or wounds that pass through the repair process without restoring anatomic and functional results."[1] Pressure, venous, and diabetic ulcers are the most common chronic wound etiologies. They are complex and expensive problems for patients, families, clinicians, and the health care system. The etiology of these lesions and the most effective treatments for them are often debated.

Why this Pocket Guide?

Most wounds heal in 2 to 4 weeks without special care. Until 30 years ago, little attention was given to the wound repair process, the ideal environment to stimulate wound repair, and dressing materials to create and maintain that environment. Now that the aging population is increasing and more patients survive grave illnesses and chronic diseases, there are more nonhealing wounds. Chronic wounds differ from acute wounds; exactly how they differ is not yet clear. They require labor-intensive multidisciplinary care and specific management protocols. Most wound healing principles, considered radical in the early 1970s, are now well accepted. There are a growing number of wound care specialists in clinical settings, laboratories, and industry. This Pocket Guide integrates the work of leading clinicians and researchers. The authors represent the multidisciplinary collaboration required to achieve optimal wound repair.

How to Use This Pocket Guide

This Pocket Guide is intended as a first-line problem-solving and treatment guide for safe and cost-effective management of chronic wounds. It is not intended as a definitive source of information on wound closure and repair. The Pocket Guide will be updated as required by research, product development, and continuing clinical experience.

1. Lazarus G, et al. Definitions and guidelines for assessment and evaluation of healing. Archives of Dermatology 1994;130:489-93.

Uninterrupted Wound Repair

Wound repair begins the moment tissue is injured. The healing process involves several predictable stages, which are best summarized in this diagram.

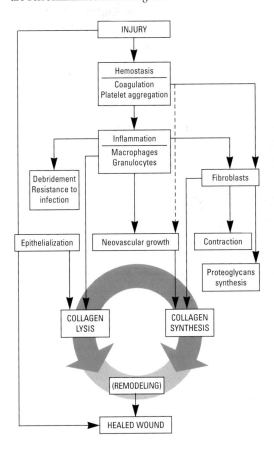

Maklebust J, Sieggreen M. Pressure ulcers: guidelines for prevention and nursing management, 2nd ed. Springhouse, PA: Springhouse Corporation; 1996: 31.

Regardless of a wound's origin, the same repair sequence must be completed. An acute wound, such as surgical incision, in a healthy middle-aged person may be expected to complete the process in a more rapid and orderly manner than a wound dehiscence in a compromised patient or a pressure ulcer in an elderly malnourished individual. The stages of chronic wound repair may not follow the sequence of an acute wound.

During the first 2 weeks of healing, an acute wound regains one-third to one-half of the skin's original strength. A wound regains nearly 80% of tensile strength after 3 months. The maturation, or remodeling, phase of healing continues for a year or more, but wounds never regain more than 80% of tensile strength. Thus, care must be taken to protect healed areas from reinjury, particularly in the first 3 months after trauma.

Elimination of exogenous and endogenous impediments to wound repair and meticulous local care are required for humane and cost-effective patient care and satisfactory treatment outcomes.

Factors Complicating Wound Repair

This chapter is intended to provide the reader with a skeletal outline of factors that might impair healing. Infection, nutrition, and aging are emphasized in other sections. The patient's overall medical status and results of a complete history and physical must be used as a reference when considering complicating factors.

Medications

The following drugs may affect wound repair:
- steroids
- antiprostaglandins
- immunosuppressants
- antineoplastics
- anticoagulants.

The patient's general medical status and concomitant medications and doses must be considered when determining effects of drugs on healing.

Aging

Factors affecting repair in the aged include but are not limited to:

- delayed cellular activity
- decreased wound breaking strength
- decreased barrier properties
- diminished biosynthetic activity
- delayed collagen remodeling and contraction
- decreased vascularity.

Although caution is suggested in treating the elderly, particularly those with friable skin, not all aged individuals have decreased ability to heal. Variations in medical status and health allow many elderly to heal as well as the younger population. Surgeries are frequently performed on the elderly without problems with healing.

When treating the elderly:

- exercise caution when using adhesives and tapes on friable skin
- avoid frequent scrubs
- avoid irritating and cytoxic agents.

For a more detailed explanation, see Chapter 6, Skin and the Aging Process.

Other Complicating Factors

Wound repair may be complicated by numerous factors both intrinsic and extrinsic. The reader is encouraged to carefully review the patient's medical status and records when determining the most appropriate form of therapy. The following is a list of miscellaneous factors that also need to be considered:

- immunosuppressive diseases
- cytotoxic cleansers, dressings, and agents
- radiation therapy
- patient's environment
- lack of attention to primary etiology of wound (i.e., inadequate pressure relief, inappropriate shoe gear, inadequate compression with venous disease) and poor patient care

- patient noncompliance
- inappropriate wound care
- nutritional status.

Note: When a wound shows no response to treatment after 2 weeks, the patient's medical and wound status need to be reevaluated. When there are no new findings regarding medical status, a different wound care product should be selected.

Surgical Indications

The most important goal in wound care is rapid and lasting closure. The question is, when should a patient be referred for surgery? There is not enough space in this pocket guide for a full discussion of the complex topic of when to refer a wound for surgical intervention. Below is an anagram that introduces some of the issues that affect that decision:

No Healing

N ecrotic tissue

O steomyelitis

H idden sinus tracts and tunnels

E schar (not removable by minor sharp debridement or dressing)

A bscess and arterial insufficiency

L arge defects too big to close by secondary intention

I schemia

N onhealing wound in spite of appropriate aggressive treatment for 30 to 45 days

G raft-ready wound beds and wound beds with tendon and bone exposed

Chapter 2

PATIENT AND WOUND EVALUATION

2

Patient Evaluation

Assessment of the patient's medical and physical status is imperative to achieve successful wound closure. This includes but is not limited to:

- thorough review of systems
- review of all medications
- review of all prior and current treatment modalities
- patient's awareness of the problem
- patient's external environment
- nutritional status.

Wound Evaluation

Evaluation and documentation includes determination of:

- etiology
- infection versus contamination
- undermining of sinus tracts
- quantity and quality of exudate
- underlying structures (muscle, tendons, bone)
- phase of healing
- chronicity
- response to previous treatment.

Note the status of the wound bed and the surrounding tissue. Color, odor, and exudate are all indications of wound status. Odor is best evaluated after a wound has been cleaned with sterile water or saline. Foul odor may result from accumulation of wound exudate, necrotic tissue, and dressing by-products, especially after the use of occlusive dressings. Wound color may indicate stage of repair. Common examples of appearance are:

red–reepithelializing	bright red with indications of superficial cell migration
red–granulating	bright or true red with islands of granulation tissue

red–chronic	red but no indication of granulation
red–dusky	dull, gray or dark red without signs of granulation, with or without signs of localized ischemia
yellow–granulating	areas of fibrotic tissue with areas of granulating tissue; no necrotic tissue present
yellow–chronic	areas of fibrotic tissue without areas of granulation
yellow–ischemic	fibrotic tissue with signs of ischemia or tissue necrosis
black–dry	black or brown, dry, desiccated eschar
black–wet	wet gangrenous appearance
black–mixed	areas of necrotic tissue present with areas of yellow and/or red tissue

Note: Fibrin (fibrotic tissue) is usually not categorized as "healthy" or "unhealthy."

Documentation

Include these descriptors in the initial documentation of a wound:

- location
- surface dimension
- color of wound base
- presence of necrotic tissue (amount and color)
- depth and tissue layers involved
- exudate (amount, color, odor)
- condition of surrounding skin
- undermining
- clinical signs of infection. (For a more detailed explanation, see Chapter 4, Microbiology.)

Wounds may be measured in a linear fashion and described as "3 cm x 5 cm" or traced on an acetate measuring guide. Tracings enable more accurate comparison of change in wound perimeter over time. Numerous companies provide small acetate sheets at no charge. Many clinicians add photographic documentation.

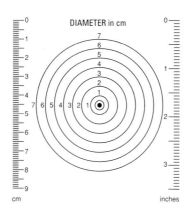

Illustration is one-half of actual size.

Measure wound depth by inserting a cotton-tipped applicator to the base of the wound, being careful not to damage underlying structures. Then measure the length of the cotton-tipped applicator that was in the wound.

Undermining, which is defined as skin overhanging a dead space, should be measured with a cotton-tipped applicator. When sinus tracts are suspected, they should be probed gently with a cotton-tipped applicator or a small red rubber catheter to determine their length.

A photograph of the wound is the most reliable documentation. Serial photographs provide objective evaluation of wound healing. A rubber stamp or standardized progress note facilitates documentation:

Wound/Pressure Ulcer Status

Date	*8/29/98*
Location	*right trochanter*
Size	*4 cm x 6 cm*
Depth	*0.75 cm*
Undermining	*1 cm from 5 to 7 o'clock position*
Wound Base	*50% yellow slough and 50% red beefy granular tissue*
Exudate	*serosanguineous*
Odor	*none*
Current Treatment	*calcium alginate every day*
Signature	*James Jones, MD, or Mary Smith, RN*

Accurate documentation enables critical evaluation of the wound healing process and helps to protect clinicians against litigation. The key to future research in the pathophysiology of chronic wounds and in therapeutic efficacy depends on precise reporting of incidence and types of chronic wounds and the use of consistent terminology.

Staging of Pressure Ulcers

Classification systems are used to describe the severity of burns, skin ulcers, congenital anomalies, and neoplasms. In many cases these staging systems have prognostic value and, in some instances, reimbursement value. Complete description and classification are essential components of the diagnostic and therapeutic process.

The National Pressure Ulcer Advisory Panel has defined this classification system for pressure ulcers:

Stage I	Observable pressure-related alteration of intact skin whose indicators as compared to an adjacent or opposite area on the body may include changes in one or more of the following: skin temperature (warmth or coolness), tissue consistency (firm or boggy feel), and/or sensation (pain, itching). The ulcer appears as a defined area of persistent redness in lightly pigmented skin, whereas in darker skin tones, the ulcer may appear with persistent red, blue, or purple hues.
Stage II	Partial-thickness skin loss involving epidermis and/or dermis. The ulcer is superficial and presents as an abrasion, blister, or shallow crater.
Stage III	Full-thickness skin loss involving damage or necrosis of subcutaneous tissue that may extend down to, but not through, underlying fascia. The ulcer presents clinically as a deep crater with or without undermining of adjacent tissue.
Stage IV	Full-thickness skin loss with extensive destruction, tissue necrosis, or damage to muscle, bone, or supporting structures (e.g., tendon, joint capsule).

9

Notes:

Microbiology

The role of bacteria in wound repair is unclear. Chronic wounds are known to be contaminated; however, the degree of contamination and the distinction between contamination and infection are difficult to determine clinically. Wound appearance can be misleading; one must rely on other signs of wound infection. One should also consider variables such as the nature of the organism, nature of the wound, and nature of the host's defense mechanisms.[1]

Indicators of Contamination Are:

- periwound erythema
- inflammation
- nonpurulent drainage
- malodorous wound prior to cleaning
- multiple organisms present on swab culture.

These same signs may be present in an infected wound.

Established Signs of Infection Are:

- elevated body temperature
- cellulitis
- purulent drainage
- wet gangrene
- increased leukocytosis
- persistently malodorous wound
- greater than 10^5 organisms per gram of tissue.

Note: The number of organisms per gram of tissue is a valid sign of infection when accompanied by other clinical signs of infection.

1. Thomson PD, Smith DJ Jr. What is infection? Amer J Surg 1994;167(1A Suppl): 7S-11S.

Other Indicators May Be:

- pain
- swelling
- redness
- inflammation
- heat.

Swab cultures are of questionable value, as multiple bacteria are often present in wound fluid and wound surface, particularly when occlusive dressings have been used. Surface organisms do not correlate well with number and types of organisms present in the tissue. Take a swab culture only when clinical signs of infection are present and adhere to the following directions. This is only a qualitative means of determining organisms present.

Swab Culture Technique for Accurate Results

- Thoroughly clean the wound with sterile saline or water prior to culturing.
- Avoid touching the wound surface with hands, gloves, or any other object.
- Swab the wound with a sterile calcium alginate or rayon swab. Do not use a cotton-tipped swab.
- Swab the wound surface for 30 seconds using a 10-point coverage.
- Avoid touching and swabbing wound margins and periwound surface.
- Place culture swab in appropriate container immediately.
- Order aerobic and anaerobic cultures.
- Send culture swab to laboratory immediately. Delays in plating may alter the results.

A punch biopsy or a needle aspiration biopsy provides a more accurate indication of the infecting organisms. These procedures should be performed by qualified and experienced clinicians. An infectious disease specialist is a valuable asset to the wound care team.

Nutrition

Optimal nutritional status is essential for every patient with a wound. About 50% of patients hospitalized on medical/surgical units of U.S. teaching hospitals suffer from protein-calorie malnutrition. Nutritional status often deteriorates during the hospital stay. Patients discharged from the hospital with open wounds are likely to have questionable nutritional status and need careful attention to nutrition if their wounds are to heal.

Nutritional Assessment

Assessing patients for signs of malnutrition is extremely important. Certain patients are at especially high risk.

Table 5.1

Patients at High Risk for Malnutrition

Historical factors present on admission:
- Patients weighing less than 80% of ideal body weight
- Patients having lost more than 10% of usual body weight in the past 6 months
- Alcoholic patients
- Elderly patients
- Patients with malabsorption syndrome
- Patients on hemodialysis

Factors to note during hospitalization:
- Poor intake
- Nothing by mouth for 3 to 5 days
- Loss of more than 10% of usual body weight
- Obesity
- Multiple trauma and burns (increased nutritional needs)
- Short-bowel syndrome, fistulas, and draining wounds (patients with increased nutrient losses)

Obese patients are often erroneously felt to benefit from calorie restriction during an acute illness. The truth is, given such stressors as trauma or sepsis, obese patients are quite susceptible to protein-calorie malnutrition and resultant poor wound healing despite an obese appearance. Numerous methods of assessing nutritional status have been advocated. Height and weight compared with ideal body weight for height can be a useful indicator of baseline nutritional status. The Metropolitan Life Insurance tables are a good reference for ideal body weight. The 1959 tables are still preferred by many clinicians.

Table 5.2

Weight-Height Reference Chart (Adults)*

Height (no shoes)	Reference Weight Women		Reference Weight Men	
Feet/inches	lb	kg	lb	kg
4'10"	101	46	-	-
4'11"	104	47	-	-
5'0"	107	49	-	-
5'1"	110	50	-	-
5'2"	113	51	124	56
5'3"	116	53	127	58
5'4"	120	54	130	59
5'5"	123	56	133	60
5'6"	128	58	137	62
5'7"	132	60	141	64
5'8"	136	62	145	66
5'9"	140	63	149	68
5'10"	144	65	153	69
5'll"	148	67	158	71
6'0"	152	69	162	74
6'1"	-	-	167	76
6'2"	-	-	171	78
6'3"	-	-	176	80
6'4"	-	-	181	82

*Data adapted from Metropolitan Life Insurance Company: 1959.

Table 5.3 provides a quick screen to identify patients who are at risk for poor wound healing.

Table 5.3

Short Screen for Protein-Calorie Malnutrition

History
- Recent weight loss, particularly greater than 10% of usual weight

Physical Examination
- Patients weighing less than 85% of ideal body weight
- Easy hair pluckability*
- Edema

Laboratory
- Low serum albumin level (less than 3.5 g/dl).

* Tested by grasping a lock of hair on the top of the head firmly between the thumb and forefinger. An abnormal result is an average of three or more hairs easily and painlessly removed with a firm tug.

The items listed are those most indicative of protein-calorie malnutrition. The edema seen in patients with protein-calorie malnutrition is due to low serum colloid osmotic pressure with resultant accumulation of interstitial fluid. Wound edema can impair healing by increasing the distance oxygen and other nutrients must travel to reach the cells and by inhibiting movement of cellular waste products, causing their build up around the wound. Edema also results in weight gain and can cause the clinician to believe erroneously that a patient's weight is stable when lean body mass is decreasing. Although no one factor is indicative of malnutrition, the more factors present, the higher the suspicion of malnutrition.

Serum protein levels have long been used as indicators of visceral protein stores. Albumin is the most well studied. A serum albumin level of less than 3.5 g/dl indicates that nutritional status should be assessed. A level less than 3.0 g/dl is certainly correlated with poor patient outcomes. Protein-calorie malnutrition has a high mortality. Once the clinician identifies hypoalbuminemia, edema, and easy hair-pluckability, the patient is in need of urgent, intensive nutritional intervention. It is preferable to implement optimal nutritional intervention much earlier in the course of wound healing and prevent this serious complication.

These formulas can be used to estimate the protein and calorie needs of a patient.

Table 5.4

Estimating Nutritional Needs for Patients with Wounds

Daily Caloric Needs:

1.2 - 1.5 x BEE (Basal Energy Expenditure)

Harris-Benedict equations for BEE:
Women: BEE = 655.1 + 9.56W + 1.85H - 4.68A
Men: BEE = 66.47 + 13.75W + 5.0H - 6.76A
(W = weight in kilograms; H = height in centimeters; A = age in years)

Daily Protein Needs:

1.5 x W

Calorie counts, including an assessment of protein intake, are necessary to judge the adequacy of protein-calorie repletion. To be sure of protein requirements, collect a 24-hour blood urea nitrogen (BUN). Protein losses = [24-hour BUN (grams) + 4] x 6.25. The 4 is an estimate of the unmeasured nitrogen lost in the urine, sweat, and stool. The 6.25 converts nitrogen to dietary protein (6.25 g protein/g nitrogen). Protein losses may be higher in patients with burns and heavily draining wounds.

If dietary intake is not sufficient to meet calculated needs, nutritional supplementation should be initiated. Tube feeding is the route of choice if the gut works. A high-protein, lactose-free formula should be selected and begun slowly (50 ml/hour). The rate can be increased every 6 to 8 hours until the patient's needs are being met. Gastric residuals should be checked before each increase in rate and should show less than 50 ml in the stomach. Dilution of the tube feeding is not helpful. The rate should be slowed if the patient has any problems tolerating the feeding. Parenteral nutrition can be extremely helpful in supplementing an inadequate oral intake. Hospitalized patients with severe stress and protein-calorie malnutrition should receive total parenteral nutrition (TPN) until their serum albumin levels have improved. The bowel of a patient with protein-calorie malnutrition may be edematous, which may result in malabsorption and diarrhea if tube feeding is begun before the serum albumin levels have improved. TPN can be gradually tapered as tube feeding or oral intake becomes adequate.

Many nutrients are thought to be important in the healing process.

Table 5.5

Nutrients Important in Wound Healing

Nutrient	Wound Healing Function	Result of Deficiency
Proteins	Wound repair Clotting factor production White blood cell production and migration Cell-mediated bacterial killing Fibroblast proliferation Neovascularization Collagen synthesis Epithelial cell proliferation Wound remodeling	Poor wound healing Hypoalbuminemia Edema Lymphopenia Impaired cellular immunity
Carbohydrates	Supply cellular energy Spare protein	Use visceral and muscle proteins for energy
Fats	Supply cellular energy Supply essential fatty acids Manufacture of cell membranes Prostaglandins production	Poor wound healing

Table 5.5 *(continued)*

Nutrient	Wound Healing Function	Result of Deficiency
Vitamin A	Collagen synthesis Epithelialization	Poor wound healing
Vitamin C	Membrane integrity	Scurvy Poor wound healing Capillary fragility
Zinc	Cell proliferation Cofactor for many enzymes	Slow wound healing Alteration in taste Anorexia

Vitamin and mineral assays are useful to confirm suspected deficiencies. There is evidence that, in the presence of deficiencies, but not in their absence, vitamin C and zinc supplementation may aid wound healing. The only nutritional supplement appropriately prescribed empirically, other than those to attain an adequate intake of protein and calories, is a daily high-potency multivitamin, multimineral supplement for nursing home patients and community-dwelling elderly patients with chronic wounds. Many of these patients have been found to be deficient in numerous vitamins and minerals, so a daily high-potency multivitamin, multimineral supplement is reasonable as well as low-cost and low-risk. Additional empiric vitamin therapy is prescribed frequently, but it has not been shown to be necessary, may be costly, and can cause adverse effects such as nausea and anorexia with zinc or toxicity with high doses of vitamin A.

Proper assessment of nutritional status and nutritional interventions to meet the protein, calorie, vitamin, and mineral needs of patients with wounds cannot be overemphasized in wound healing.

SKIN AND THE AGING PROCESS

6

Skin of the Elderly

It is well recognized that the skin of the elderly differs in many ways from that of a younger person. Although physiologic response to aging varies, certain characteristics are inherent to the aging process.

To understand gerontodermatologic changes and the effects they have on delayed wound healing, it is important to review what is normal so that the changes that take place can be understood.

An average person's skin would probably measure over 20 sq ft (about 2 m²) if it were laid out flat, and it would weigh about 5½ lb (over 2 kg). Skin on an average weighs about twice as much as the brain. It is commonly called "the body's biggest organ" and is the only organ that is completely exposed to the external environment.

Skin is an all-purpose covering. It is waterproof in both directions. It keeps water out and, more importantly, keeps water in.

At its thickest (back, soles of feet, and palms), skin measures approximately ⅛". At its thinnest (eyelids), it measures approximately ¹⁄₂₅".

Skin is made up of three layers:
- epidermis
- dermis
- subcutis.

Epidermis

The epidermis is the top, or uppermost, skin layer. It is no thicker than a page in a book. The epidermis constantly replaces itself. Every hour you shed about 1 million dead skin cells. At the end of each month you have an almost completely new epidermis. Most "house dust" is thought to be dead skin that has rubbed off the bodies of people.

The epidermis is subdivided into three parts:

- stratum corneum (top layer)
- stratum spinosum (middle layer)
- stratum germinativum (bottom layer).

The stratum corneum, or the horny layer, is somewhat acidic and is referred to as the acid mantle. It is the only major physical barrier to the environment. It effectively prevents the penetration of most environmental substances that come in contact with skin or are applied to it. Only substances possessing a molecular size smaller than the size of water molecules can readily penetrate this epidermal barrier.

The stratum spinosum is called the prickle cell layer. This is the thickest of the epidermal layers. The cells in the stratum spinosum are known as squamous cells. Essentially, squamous cells are basal cells that have matured and migrated upward with the epidermis.

The stratum germinativum is called the basal layer and continually gives birth to new cells. It contains basal cells and melanocytes. Usually one out of six cells in the basal layer is a melanocyte. These produce melanin, which is responsible for imparting color to skin.

Dermis

The dermis, the second layer of skin, is under the epidermis. It contains collagen and elastic fibers, which are complex proteins responsible for the support and elasticity of the skin. They enable skin to regain its shape after being stretched or pulled. The dermis contains blood vessels that bring nutrients, oxygen, and water to the skin; nerve endings that sense touch, heat, cold, and pain; and sweat glands and oil glands that help to keep skin supple and waterproof. Skin nutrition and oxygenation are supplied by the numerous tiny arteries, veins, and capillaries coursing upward through the dermis. These vessels branch from larger vessels situated more deeply in the body. Incredibly, each square inch of the dermis houses 15" of small, nutrient-providing blood vessels. Their constriction and dilation, in response to extremes of heat and cold, are responsible for keeping the body temperature constant. These small blood vessels also keep the skin healthy and viable and remove metabolic waste materials.

Subcutis

The subcutis is the fatty layer that helps skin look smooth.

Gerontodermatologic Changes

With aging, the normal physiology of skin is altered. The following reviews the gerontodermatologic changes to each of the layers and how these changes can affect wound healing.

Changes to the Epidermis

Changes:	Results:
Thinning and flattening of the epidermis	• increased vulnerability to trauma • increased skin susceptibility to shearing stress, thereby promoting blister formation and skin tears • decreased tissue barrier properties • impairment of the skin's extremely important barrier functions, causing problems by allowing certain drugs and irritants to be more easily absorbed
Decreased epidermal proliferation	• the production of new skin cells slows down, and the epidermis cannot replace itself as quickly • decreased wound contraction • delayed cellular migration and proliferation
Cells in the horny layer lose elastin fibers	• the skin of older people is like a worn rubber band – it does not snap back fast or have much elasticity

Changes to the Dermis

Changes:	Results:
Atrophy of the dermis	• underlying tissues more vulnerable to injury • increased rate of wound dehiscence • decreased wound contraction
Decreased vascularity of the dermis	• easy bruisability and susceptibility to injury • decreased skin temperature • increased vulnerability to trauma • decreased wound capillary growth • increased rate of wound dehiscence
Changes to and loss of collagen and elastic fibers	• underlying tissues are more vulnerable to injury • decreased tensile strength • delayed collagen remodeling
Decrease in number of oil and sweat glands	• skin not as moist or well lubricated
Vascular response is compromised	• impaired cutaneous immune and inflammatory responses • reduced ability to clear foreign materials and fluids • decreased wound capillary growth • altered metabolic response
Nerve endings become abnormal	• altered or reduced sensation

Changes to the Subcutis

Changes:	Results:
Fragility	• easy bruisability and tearing of the skin • loss of cushion effect • skin no longer as thick

Incontinence Care

Incontinent immobile patients are at greater risk for developing pressure ulcers. Fecal incontinence has been associated with the development of pressure ulcers. Aggressive, preventive skin care for all incontinent patients is urgently needed. The essential components in most incontinence skin care protocols are cleansers, moisturizers, and barrier creams, ointments, or films.

Perineal Cleansers

Select a perineal wash with surfactants and humectants. Perineal care should be done in the morning, evening, after bowel movements, and as needed. Avoid soap and detergents, such as sodium laurel sulfate, that may cause drying or irritation of the skin.

Moisturizers

Moisturizers come in the form of lotions or creams. They should not have a high alcohol content, which is drying to the skin. Moisturizers should be rubbed in until they vanish to preserve moisture in the skin.

Barrier Creams, Ointments, and Films

A water-repellent barrier cream, ointment, or film should be used if a patient has continuous incontinence or wound drainage. Product selection should be made according to the needs of the patient and the staff. Some patients with periodic incontinence benefit most from a perineal wash followed by a moisturizing agent. Others, with continuous drainage, may need only a cleanser and a barrier, unless they have very dry skin that needs to be moisturized before applying the barrier. When patients have denuded skin, it is helpful to dust the open area lightly with a carboxymethylcellulose powder, which is commonly used in ostomy care. Such a powder absorbs the surface moisture sufficiently to allow application of a cream or ointment.

When patients have suspected or obvious fungal rashes, a prescription antifungal agent is required. Antifungal products are available in powders or creams. An over-the-counter antifungal powder may be used prophylactically for patients taking antibiotics and for patients with mild rashes characterized by diffuse redness and itching.

Pressure Ulcers

The pathophysiology of pressure ulcers is not fully under-stood because the ulcer represents a destructive process that has already occurred. It has been established that pressure, friction, shear, and moisture damage skin and subcutaneous tissue. Immobility, inactivity, malnutrition, fecal and urinary incontinence, and a decreased level of consciousness are known risk factors associated with the development of pressure ulcers.

Early Intervention

Early intervention refers to treatment prescribed for patients who are likely to develop pressure ulcers as determined by a risk assessment tool. Early intervention requires:
* adequate pressure reduction/relief
* frequent repositioning
* attention to nutritional status
* aggressive and gentle perineal care
* protective devices that lift heels off the bed padding for ankles and knees.

Treatment

When a pressure ulcer occurs, these principles should guide treatment:[1]
* Relieve pressure.
* Debride necrotic tissue.
* Maintain a clean, moist wound environment.
* Correct contributing factors, e.g., malnutrition, diarrhea, urinary incontinence.

1. Bergstrom N, et al. Treatment of pressure ulcers. Clinical Practice Guideline, No. 15. AHCPR Publication No. 95-0652. Rockville, MD: Agency for Health Care Policy and Research, Public Health Service, U.S. Department of Health and Human Services; 1994.

Relieve Pressure

The most important component to pressure relief is the duration and intensity of pressure. A clinician must know the surface on which a patient lies and be aware of the angle at which the body is positioned. Support surfaces are described in Chapter 13, Support Surfaces.

- Do not position patients with the head of the bed at greater than a 30-degree angle for an extended period of time. This position allows shearing forces to crimp and occlude blood flow to the sacral or ischial areas.

- Use a bed pillow or special cushion to provide adequate pressure reduction for patients who are seated for prolonged periods. Encourage or assist weight shifts in the chair every 15 minutes.

- Reposition immobile patients in bed every 2 hours and more frequently if they have been determined to be at high risk or if an ulcer is present.

- Patients should be maintained at a 30-degree angle rather than logrolled from side to side. Do not position patients with a pressure ulcer directly on the ulcer, unless they are on a pressure relief surface.

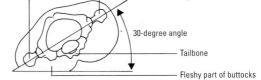

Maklebust J, Sieggreen M. Pressure ulcers: guidelines for prevention and nursing management, 2nd ed. Springhouse, PA: Springhouse Corporation; 1996: 78.

Debride Necrotic Tissue

Use one of these three methods to debride necrotic tissue.

1. **Sharp Debridement –** Sharp debridement down to the level of viable tissue is the most effective, economical means of removing necrotic tissue. Before performing sharp debridement check your state's practice act to determine if your license allows you to do this.

2. Enzymatic Debridement – Enzymatic debriding agents, which are ordered by prescription only, devitalize necrotic tissue. Some agents destroy healthy tissue. Apply enzymatic debriding agents to the wound 1 or 2 times a day.

3. Autolytic Debridement – Autolytic debridement allows necrotic tissue to self-digest from enzymes present in the wound fluids. The following dressing types promote autolytic debridement:

- **Transparent Film Dressings** – Change dressings every 24 to 72 hours to remove liquefied necrotic material. Irrigate the wound thoroughly with normal saline and inspect the wound bed.

- **Amorphous Hydrogel Dressings** – Change dressings every 24 to 72 hours (or every 1 to 7 days) per package insert to remove liquefied necrotic material. Irrigate the wound thoroughly with normal saline and inspect the wound bed. Hydrogels are more effective for debriding dry and low exudate wounds.

- **Hydrocolloid Wafer Dressings** – Change dressings every 2 to 7 days per package insert to remove liquefied necrotic material. Irrigate the wound thoroughly with normal saline and inspect the wound bed.

- **Calcium Alginates** – Change dressings every 24 hours per package insert to remove liquefied necrotic material. Irrigate the wound thoroughly with normal saline and inspect the wound bed.

Wound Cleansing

Use normal saline or a nonionic surfactant wound cleanser to remove wound debris and dressing material residue at every dressing change. Harsh disinfecting agents are cytotoxic to granulation tissue and should not be used in wound care. Irrigate wounds with a 19-gauge needle or angiocath and a 35-ml syringe, which will apply enough force to remove debris.

Observable pressure-related alteration of intact skin (see page 9 for indicators).

Objectives
- Cover
- Protect

Product
Lubricating spray, ointment, or moisturizer

Frequency of Use
Two or three times daily.

Procedure
- Position patient off affected area.
- Gently clean affected area. Blot dry.
- Apply small amount of lubricating spray, ointment, or moisturizer and smooth into skin.

Note: Vigorous massage is not recommended for reddened skin. It may stimulate undesired blood flow to the area and cause further damage to fragile tissue.

Product
Transparent film dressing

Frequency of Use
Every 5 to 7 days or when reddened area has resolved. Change if patient movement dislodges dressing.

Procedure
- Position patient off affected area.
- Select a dressing that allows at least a 2" margin of intact skin beyond the reddened area.
- Apply a skin sealant to all intact skin to be covered with dressing. Allow to dry until slick.
- Apply dressing, avoiding tension and skin wrinkling that would cause further damage.
- Write date of application and initials of applier directly on the dressing.

Note: When using transparent film dressings over the coccyx, do not pull dressing from one buttock to the other. This may create tension on the skin. Also, bridging the gluteal cleft interferes with the dressing's adherence. Instead, apply the dressing in a crisscross fashion and overlap it, or begin with the application of a single piece in the center and work from left to right.

Product
Hydrocolloid wafer or semipermeable foam dressing

Frequency of Use
Every 5 to 7 days or when reddened area has resolved. Change if patient movement dislodges dressing.

Procedure
- Position patient off affected area.
- Select a dressing that allows at least a 2" margin of intact skin beyond the reddened area.
- Apply a skin sealant to all intact skin to be covered with dressing. Allow to dry until slick.
- Apply dressing, avoiding tension and skin wrinkling that would cause further damage.
- Write date of application and initials of applier directly on the dressing.

Stage II

Partial-thickness skin loss involving epidermis and/or dermis. The ulcer is superficial and presents clinically as a blister, abrasion, or shallow crater.

Objectives
- Cover
- Protect
- Insulate
- Absorb
- Hydrate

Stage II: Blister

Product
Transparent film dressing

Frequency of Use
Only when patient movement dislodges dressing or blister fluid is absorbed.

Procedure

- Position patient off affected area.
- Gently clean affected area. Blot dry.
- Apply skin sealant to all intact skin to be covered with transparent film dressing (including the blister). Allow to dry until slick.
- Select a dressing that allows at least a 2" margin of intact skin beyond blister.
- Apply dressing, avoiding tension and skin wrinkling that would cause further damage.
- Write date of application and initials of applier directly on the dressing.

Note: The dressing should be changed if the blister ruptures and drainage leaks out of the transparent film dressing.

Stage II: Abrasion or shallow crater with minimal drainage

Product
Transparent film dressing

Frequency of Use
Every 3 to 5 days or when wound fluid leaks out beyond dressing.

Procedure

- Position patient off affected area.
- Gently clean affected area. Blot dry.
- Apply a skin sealant to all intact skin to be covered with dressing. Allow to dry until slick.
- Select a dressing that allows at least a 2" margin of intact skin beyond the wound edge.
- Apply dressing, avoiding tension and skin wrinkling that would cause further damage.
- Write date of application and initials of applier directly on the dressing.

Note: When using transparent film dressings over the coccyx, do not pull dressing from one buttock to the other. This may create tension on the skin. Also, bridging the gluteal cleft interferes with the dressing's adherence. Instead, apply the dressing in a crisscross fashion and overlap it, or begin the application of a single piece in the center and work from left to right.

Product
Amorphous hydrogel dressing

Frequency of Use
Every 24 to 48 hours, depending on wound drainage.

Procedure
- Position patient off affected area.
- Use normal saline or a nonionic surfactant wound cleanser to clean wound.
- Blot surrounding skin dry.
- Apply skin sealant to periwound skin. Allow to dry until slick.
- Lightly coat the wound bed with amorphous hydrogel dressing.
- Cover with transparent film dressing or nonadherent dressing.
- Write date of application and initials of applier directly on the dressing.

Product
Hydrocolloid wafer dressing

Frequency of Use
Every 3 to 7 days. Change when drainage leaks out or when dressing becomes loose or soiled.

Procedure
- Position patient off affected area.
- Use normal saline or a nonionic surfactant wound cleanser to remove wound debris and dressing material residue.
- Blot surrounding skin dry.
- Apply skin sealant to periwound skin. Allow to dry until slick.
- Select a wafer that extends at least 2" beyond the wound area or cut a piece to fit from a larger wafer.
- Peel protective backing off wafer and center the dressing over wound.
- Write date of application and initials of applier directly on the dressing.

Note: Apply strips of tape around the perimeter of the wafer in the sacral area or on heels and elbows. A skin sealant should be applied to skin that will be covered by tape. Wound fluid may have a disturbing appearance and odor when dressings are changed. Evaluate the wound's condition after thorough, gentle irrigation. Wounds with necrotic tissue may appear deeper and larger as nonviable tissue sloughs.

Stage II: Abrasion or shallow crater with moderate to heavy drainage

Product
Semipermeable foam wafer.

Frequency of Use
Every 3 to 5 days, depending on amount of exudate present or when strike through approaches the edges of the dressing. Individualize the frequency of dressing change based on the amount of wound drainage and package insert.

Procedure
- Position patient off affected area.
- Use normal saline or a nonionic surfactant wound cleanser to clean wound.
- Blot surrounding skin dry.
- Apply skin sealant to periwound skin. Allow to dry until slick.
- Place semipermeable foam dressing over the wound. If needed, tape margins with nonaggressive tape. Self-adhesive fabric tape also may be used to secure dressing.
- Write date of application and initials of applier directly on the dressing.

Product
Calcium alginate

Frequency of Use
Every 24 to 48 hours per package insert. Individualize frequency of dressing change depending on the amount of wound drainage.

Procedure

- Position patient off affected area.
- Use normal saline or a nonionic surfactant wound cleanser to remove wound debris and dressing material residue.
- Blot surrounding skin dry.
- Apply skin sealant to periwound skin. Allow to dry until slick.
- Apply calcium alginate dressing to the wound bed.
- Cover with absorbent gauze, nonwoven pad, or transparent film dressing.
- Secure cover dressing with hypoallergenic tape, if needed. Self-adhesive fabric tape also may be used to secure dressings.
- Write date of application and initials of applier directly on the dressing.

Note: A brownish green viscous residue may appear in the wound bed or in soiled dressings. This is probably a dressing by-product. Evaluate wound after thorough, gentle irrigation.

Stage III

Full-thickness skin loss involving damage or necrosis of subcutaneous tissue, which may extend down to, but not through, underlying fascia. The ulcer presents clinically as a deep crater with or without undermining of adjacent tissue.

Objectives

- Cover
- Protect
- Hydrate
- Insulate
- Absorb
- Clean
- Prevent infection
- Promote granulation

Shallow Stage III: Small amount of drainage

Product

Amorphous hydrogel dressing

Frequency of Use

Every 24 to 48 hours, depending on wound drainage.

Procedure

- Position patient off affected area.
- Use normal saline or a nonionic surfactant wound cleanser to clean wound.
- Blot surrounding skin dry.
- Apply skin sealant to periwound skin. Allow to dry until slick.
- Lightly coat the wound bed with amorphous hydrogel dressing.
- Cover with transparent film dressing or nonadherent dressing.
- Write date of application and initials of applier directly on the dressing.

Product

Hydrocolloid wafer dressing

Frequency of Use

Every 3 to 7 days. Change when drainage leaks out or when dressing becomes loose or soiled.

Procedure

- Position patient off affected area.
- Use normal saline or a nonionic surfactant wound cleanser to remove wound debris and dressing material residue.
- Blot surrounding skin dry.
- Apply skin sealant to periwound skin. Allow to dry until slick.
- Select a wafer that extends at least 2" beyond the wound area or cut a piece to fit from a larger wafer.
- Peel protective backing off the wafer and center the dressing over wound.
- Write date of application and initials of applier directly on the dressing.

Note: Apply strips of tape around the perimeter of the wafer in the sacral area or on heels and elbows. A skin sealant should be applied to skin that will be covered by tape. Wound fluid may have a disturbing appearance and odor when dressings are changed. Evaluate the wound's condition after thorough, gentle irrigation. Wounds with necrotic tissue may appear deeper and larger as nonviable tissue sloughs.

Deep Stage III: Small amount of drainage

Product
Impregnated hydrogel dressing

Frequency of Use
Every 24 to 48 hours depending on wound drainage.

Procedure
- Position patient off affected area.
- Use normal saline or a nonionic surfactant wound cleanser to clean wound.
- Blot surrounding skin dry.
- Apply skin sealant to periwound skin. Allow to dry until slick.
- Lightly pack wound with impregnated hydrogel dressing.
- If the wound has tunneling, loosely pack with impregnated hydrogel dressing, ribbon gauze moistened with normal saline, or an amorphous hydrogel dressing.
- Cover with transparent film dressing or nonadherent dressing.
- Write date of application and initials of applier directly on the dressing.

Product
Hydrocolloid wafer dressing

Frequency of Use
Every 3 to 7 days. Change when drainage leaks out or when dressing becomes loose or soiled.

Procedure
- Position patient off affected area.
- Use normal saline or a nonionic surfactant wound cleanser to remove wound debris and dressing material residue.
- Blot surrounding skin dry.

- Apply skin sealant to periwound skin. Allow to dry until slick.
- Select a wafer that extends at least 2" beyond the wound area or cut a piece to fit from a larger wafer.
- Fill the cavity with a hydrocolloid gel or paste.
- Peel protective backing off wafer and center the dressing over wound.
- Write date of application and initials of applier directly on the dressing.

Note: Apply strips of tape around the perimeter of the wafer in the sacral area or on heels and elbows. A skin sealant should be applied to skin that will be covered by tape. Wound fluid may have a disturbing appearance and odor when dressings are changed. Evaluate the wound's condition after thorough, gentle irrigation. Wounds with necrotic tissue may appear deeper and larger as nonviable tissue sloughs.

Shallow Stage III: Moderate to heavy drainage

Product
Calcium alginate

Frequency of Use
Every 24 to 48 hours per package insert. Individualize frequency of dressing change depending on the wound drainage amount.

Procedure
- Position patient off affected area.
- Use normal saline or a nonionic surfactant wound cleanser to remove wound debris and dressing material residue.
- Blot surrounding skin dry.
- Apply skin sealant to periwound skin. Allow to dry until slick.
- Apply calcium alginate dressing to the wound bed.
- Cover with absorbent gauze, nonwoven pad, or transparent film dressing. If the wound has heavy drainage, cover calcium alginate with a semi-permeable foam wafer.

- Secure cover dressing with hypoallergenic tape, if needed. Self-adhesive fabric tape also may be used to secure dressings.
- Write date of application and initials of applier directly on the dressing.

Note: A brownish green viscous residue may appear in the wound bed or in soiled dressings. This is probably a dressing by-product. Evaluate wound after thorough, gentle irrigation.

Product
Semipermeable foam wafer

Frequency of Use
Every 3 to 5 days, depending on amount of exudate that is present or when strike through approaches the edges of the dressing. Individualize the frequency of dressing change based on the amount of wound drainage and package insert.

Procedure
- Position patient off affected area.
- Use normal saline or a nonionic surfactant wound cleanser to clean wound.
- Blot surrounding skin dry.
- Apply skin sealant to periwound skin. Allow to dry until slick.
- Place semipermeable foam wafer over the wound. Tape margins with nonaggressive tape, if needed. Self-adhesive fabric tape also may be used to secure dressings.
- Write date of application and initials of applier directly on the dressing.

Deep Stage III: Moderate to heavy drainage

Product
Calcium alginate or hydrofiber

Frequency of Use
Every 24 to 96 hours per package insert. Individualize frequency of dressing change depending on the wound drainage amount.

Procedure

- Position patient off affected area.
- Use normal saline or a nonionic surfactant wound cleanser to remove wound debris and dressing material residue.
- Blot surrounding skin dry.
- Apply skin sealant to periwound skin. Allow to dry until slick.
- Apply dressing to the wound cavity.
- If the wound has tunneling, pack lightly with a calcium alginate rope.
- Cover with absorbent gauze, nonwoven pad, or transparent film dressing. If the wound has heavy drainage, cover calcium alginate with a semipermeable foam wafer.
- Secure cover dressing with hypoallergenic tape, if needed. Self-adhesive fabric tape also may be used to secure dressings.
- Write date of application and initials of applier directly on the dressing.

Note: A brownish green viscous residue may appear in the wound bed or in soiled dressings. This is probably a dressing by-product. Evaluate wound after thorough, gentle irrigation.

Product

Semipermeable foam cavity.

Frequency of Use

Every 3 to 5 days, depending on amount of exudate that is present or when strike through approaches the edges of the dressing. Individualize the frequency of dressing change based on the amount of wound drainage and package insert.

Procedure

- Position patient off affected area.
- Use normal saline or a nonionic surfactant wound cleanser to clean wound.
- Blot surrounding skin dry.
- Apply skin sealant to periwound skin. Allow to dry until slick.

- Place semipermeable foam cavity into the wound cavity.
- Cover semipermeable foam cavity with semipermeable foam wafer or absorbent cover. If absorbent cover dressing is used, no cover or tape is needed.
- Tape margins with nonaggressive tape, if needed. Self-adhesive fabric tape also may be used to secure dressings.
- Write date of application and initials of applier directly on the dressing.

Stage IV

Full-thickness skin loss with extensive destruction, tissue necrosis, or damage to muscle, bone, or supporting structures (e.g., tendon, joint capsule).

Objectives
- Cover
- Protect
- Hydrate
- Insulate
- Absorb
- Clean
- Prevent infection
- Obliterate dead space
- Promote granulation

Shallow Stage IV: Small amount of drainage

Product
Amorphous hydrogel dressing

Frequency of Use
Every 24 to 48 hours, depending on wound drainage.

Procedure
- Position patient off affected area.
- Use normal saline or a nonionic surfactant wound cleanser to clean wound.
- Blot surrounding skin dry.
- Apply skin sealant to periwound skin. Allow to dry until slick.
- Lightly coat the wound bed with amorphous hydrogel dressing.

39

- Cover with transparent film dressing or nonadherent dressing.
- Write date of application and initials of applier directly on the dressing.

Product
Hydrocolloid wafer dressing

Frequency of Use
Every 3 to 7 days. Change when drainage leaks out or when dressing becomes loose or soiled.

Procedure
- Position patient off affected area.
- Use normal saline or a nonionic surfactant wound cleanser to remove wound debris and dressing material residue.
- Blot surrounding skin dry.
- Apply skin sealant to periwound skin. Allow to dry until slick.
- Select a wafer that extends at least 2" beyond the wound area or cut a piece to fit from a larger wafer.
- Peel protective backing off the wafer and center the dressing over wound.
- Write date of application and initials of applier directly on the dressing.

Note: Apply strips of tape around the perimeter of the wafer in the sacral area or on heels and elbows. A skin sealant should be applied to skin that will be covered by tape. Wound fluid may have a disturbing appearance and odor when dressings are changed. Evaluate the wound's condition after thorough, gentle irrigation. Wounds with necrotic tissue may appear deeper and larger as nonviable tissue sloughs.

Deep Stage IV: Small amount of drainage

Product
Impregnated hydrogel dressing.

Frequency of Use
Every 24 to 48 hours, depending on wound drainage.

Procedure

- Position patient off affected area.
- Use normal saline or a nonionic surfactant wound cleanser to clean wound.
- Blot surrounding skin dry.
- Apply skin sealant to periwound skin. Allow to dry until slick.
- Lightly pack wound with impregnated hydrogel dressing.
- If the wound has tunneling, loosely pack with impregnated hydrogel dressing, ribbon gauze moistened with normal saline, or amorphous hydrogel.
- Cover with transparent film dressing or nonadherent dressing.
- Write date of application and initials of applier directly on the dressing.

Product

Hydrocolloid wafer dressing

Frequency of Use

Every 3 to 7 days. Always change when drainage leaks out or when dressing becomes loose or soiled.

Procedure

- Position patient off affected area.
- Use normal saline or a nonionic surfactant wound cleanser to remove wound debris and dressing material residue.
- Blot surrounding skin dry.
- Apply skin sealant to periwound skin. Allow to dry until slick.
- Select a wafer that extends at least 2" beyond the wound area or cut a piece to fit from a larger wafer.
- Fill the cavity with hydrocolloid gel or paste.
- Peel protective backing off wafer and center the dressing over wound.
- Write date of application and initials of applier directly on the dressing.

Note: Apply strips of tape around the perimeter of the

*wafer in the sacral area or on heels and elbows. A skin
sealant should be applied to skin that will be covered
by tape. Wound fluid may have a disturbing appearance and odor when dressings are changed. Evaluate
the wound's condition after thorough, gentle irrigation. Wounds with necrotic tissue may appear deeper
and larger as nonviable tissue sloughs.*

Shallow Stage IV: Moderate to heavy drainage

Product
Calcium alginate

Frequency of Use
Every 24 to 48 hours per package insert. Individualize frequency of dressing change depending on the wound
drainage amount.

Procedure
- Position patient off affected area.
- Use normal saline or a nonionic surfactant wound
  cleanser to remove wound debris and dressing
  material residue.
- Blot surrounding skin dry.
- Apply skin sealant to periwound skin. Allow to dry
  until slick.
- Apply calcium alginate dressing to the wound bed.
- Cover with absorbent gauze, nonwoven pad, or
  transparent film dressing. If the wound has heavy
  drainage, cover calcium alginate with a semipermeable foam wafer.
- Secure cover dressing with hypoallergenic tape, if
  needed. Self-adhesive fabric tape also may be used
  to secure dressings.
- Write date of application and initials of applier
  directly on the dressing.

*Note: A brownish green viscous residue may appear in
the wound bed or in soiled dressings. This is probably a
dressing by-product. Evaluate wound after thorough,
gentle irrigation.*

Product
Semipermeable foam wafers

Frequency of Use

Every 3 to 5 days, depending on amount of exudate that is present or when strike through approaches the edges of the dressing. Individualize the frequency of dressing change based on the amount of wound drainage and package insert.

Procedure

- Position patient off affected area.
- Use normal saline or a nonionic surfactant wound cleanser to clean wound.
- Blot surrounding skin dry.
- Apply skin sealant to periwound skin. Allow to dry until slick.
- Place semipermeable foam wafer over the wound.
- Tape margins with nonaggressive tape, if needed. Self-adhesive fabric tape also may be used to secure dressings.
- Write date of application and initials of applier directly on the dressing.

Deep Stage IV: Moderate to heavy drainage

Product

Calcium alginate or hydrofiber

Frequency of Use

Change every 24 to 96 hours per package insert. Individualize frequency of dressing change depending on the wound drainage amount.

Procedure

- Position patient off affected area.
- Use normal saline or a nonionic surfactant wound cleanser to remove wound debris and dressing material residue.
- Blot surrounding skin dry.
- Apply skin sealant to periwound skin. Allow to dry until slick.
- Apply calcium alginate dressing to the wound cavity.
- If the wound has tunneling, pack lightly with a calcium alginate rope.
- Cover with absorbent gauze, nonwoven pad, or

transparent film dressing. If the wound has heavy drainage, cover calcium alginate with a semi-permeable foam wafer.

- Secure cover dressing with hypoallergenic tape, if needed. Self-adhesive fabric tape also may be used to secure dressings.
- Write date of application and initials of applier directly on the dressing.

Note: A brownish green viscous residue may appear in the wound bed or in soiled dressings. This is probably a dressing by-product. Evaluate wound after thorough, gentle irrigation.

Product
Semipermeable foam cavity

Frequency of Use
Every 3 to 5 days, depending on amount of exudate that is present or when strike through approaches the edges of the dressing. Individualize the frequency of dressing change based on the amount of wound drainage and package insert.

Procedure
- Position patient off affected area.
- Use normal saline or a nonionic surfactant wound cleanser to clean wound.
- Blot surrounding skin dry.
- Apply skin sealant to periwound skin. Allow to dry until slick.
- Place semipermeable foam cavity into the wound cavity.
- Cover semipermeable foam cavity with semipermeable foam wafer.
- Tape margins with nonaggressive tape, if needed. Self-adhesive fabric tape also may be used to secure dressings.
- Write date of application and initials of applier directly on the dressing.

Saline-Soaked Gauze Dressings

Saline-soaked, fluffed gauze dressings applied in wet-to-damp fashion may be used on Stages II, III, and IV pressure ulcers. They may not be cost-effective, however, in terms of nursing time, materials cost, and effect on viable tissue when allowed to dry. Wet-to-dry saline-soaked gauze dressings are a form of non-selective mechanical debridement and should be avoided.

Product
Saline-soaked gauze dressing (wet-to-damp)

Frequency of Use
Every 6 to 8 hours.

Procedure
- Position patient off affected area.
- Apply a skin sealant to all intact skin around wound that will be covered with dressing and tape. Allow to dry until slick.
- Open gauze squares (nonwoven dressing sponges) and fluff.
- Saturate with normal saline.
- Squeeze out excess moisture. Refluff.
- Pack loosely into wound. Tuck into tracts and recessed aspects of wound to serve as wick for drainage and to obliterate dead space.
- Cover with dry gauze or absorbent pad.
- Secure with hypoallergenic tape. Self-adhesive fabric tape also may be used to secure dressings.
- Write date of application and initials of applier directly on the dressing.

Note: Do not allow the dressing to dry between changes because the wound will dehydrate. If the dressing appears dry or adherent to the wound bed, saturate the dry dressing with normal saline before removing to prevent trauma to new granulation tissue.

Gauze and Silver Sulfadiazine Packing

Gauze impregnated with silver sulfadiazine may be used in Stages III and IV pressure ulcers to help decrease bacterial burden. Silver sulfadiazine-impregnated gauze is not recommended for use in heavily exuding wounds, for longer than 2 weeks, or in patients with a history of allergy or sensitivity to sulfa drugs. Silver sulfadiazine is commonly used for burns.

Product
Silver sulfadiazine-impregnated gauze

Frequency of Use
Once a day.

Procedure
- Position patient off affected area.
- Use normal saline or a nonionic surfactant wound cleanser to clean wound.
- Blot surrounding skin dry.
- Apply skin sealant to periwound skin. Allow to dry until slick.
- Open gauze squares (nonwoven dressing sponges) and fluff.
- Saturate with silver sulfadiazine.
- Squeeze out excess moisture. Refluff.
- Pack loosely into wound. Tuck into tracts and recessed aspects of wound to serve as wick for drainage and to obliterate dead space.
- Cover with a nonadherent gauze dressing.
- Tape margins with nonaggressive tape, if needed. Self-adhesive fabric tape also may be used to secure dressings.
- Write date of application and initials of applier directly on the dressing.

Note: Whenever possible, silver sulfadiazine should not be used for more than 2 weeks. Limited amount should be used. Do not place a bolus of silver sulfadiazine into wounds.

Chapter 9

LOWER EXTREMITY ULCERS

9

Venous Ulcers

Venous ulcers occur predominantly in an ambulatory population, although they also may be found on patients who use wheelchairs and other patients who are nonambulatory.

Pathophysiology

Various theories exist regarding the etiology of venous ulcers. The four most popular hypotheses are:

- calf and foot muscle pump failure
- damage secondary to white blood cell adhesion to capillaries
- pericapillary fibrin deposition
- vein damage secondary to trauma.

Healing is best expedited by:

- increasing venous return
- decreasing venous stasis (and associated edema)
- appropriate compression
- addressing the wound environment.

Characteristics

- medial lower leg and ankle (40% occurrence)
- lipodermatosclerosis
- periwound and leg hyperpigmentation
- superficial
- frequently moderate to high exudate
- pain often relieved by elevation
- commonly associated with dermatitis

Note: The other 60% of venous ulcers occur on other areas of the lower extremities, including the lateral leg and peri-ankle tissue.

Vascular Examination

A careful and accurate assessment of the patient's vascular status is essential in ruling out arterial disease in patients presenting with chronic wounds. The following noninvasive diagnostic options are available:

- manual palpation of pulses
- Doppler examination
- venous Duplex ultrasonography
- plethysmography.

Manual palpation of major vessels of the lower extremity (posterior tibial artery and dorsal artery of the foot) gives an indication of blood flow. It is often inaccurate and may reflect the examiner's own pulses. (For a more detailed explanation, see Chapter 10, Vascular Testing.)

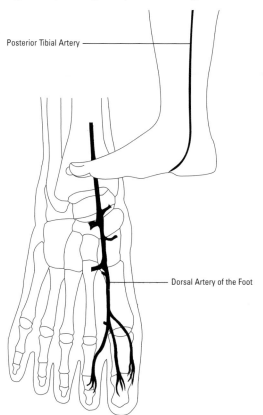

Posterior Tibial Artery

Dorsal Artery of the Foot

Wound Dressings

Many patients with venous disease are sensitive to adhesives, preservatives, and additives in products. The authors recommend avoiding the use of adhesive products, as well as those with high contents of propylene glycol, parabens, wool alcohols, and other sensitizing agents, on patients with venous disease.

Preulceration

Discoloration of skin. With venous ulcers, this may present an area of white atrophy or dermatitis occurring before a complete skin break.

Product
Hydrogels and hydrocolloids

Frequency of Use
Every 3 to 7 days

Procedure
- Clean the area with normal saline or skin cleanser.
- Blot skin dry.
- Apply dressing as indicated by the package insert.

Product
Semipermeable foam wafers

Frequency of Use
Every 3 to 7 days

Procedure
- Clean area with normal saline.
- Blot skin dry.
- Apply dressing.
- Avoid adhesives. Use gauze wrap to hold in place.

Partial-Thickness and Full-Thickness

Excluding exposure of tendon, capsule, muscle, or bone.

Product
Hydrogels and hydrocolloids

Frequency of Use
Every 1 to 3 days.

Procedure

• Same as described for Preulceration.

Product

Semipermeable foam wafers

Frequency of Use

Every 1 to 2 days.

Procedure

• Same as described for Preulceration.

Product

Calcium alginates

Frequency of Use

Once to twice per day

Procedure

• Clean area with normal saline.
• Blot skin dry.
• Apply dressing.
• Fix dressing in place with nonadherent material.

Product

Hydrofibers (moderate to heavy exudate)

Frequency of Use

Every 3 to 7 days under compression

Procedure

• Clean area with normal saline.
• Blot skin dry.
• Apply dressing according to package insert.
• Cover with a hydorcolloid dressing.

Product

Absorbent cover dressing (moderate to heavy exudate)

Frequency of Use

Every 3 to 7 days under compression

Procedure

• Clean area with normal saline.
• Blot skin dry.
• Apply dressing according to package insert.

Full-Thickness

With exposure of tendon, capsule, muscle, or bone. Avoid adhesive coverings.

Product
Amorphous hydrogels

Frequency of Use
Once to twice daily, if wound needs hydration

Procedure
- Same as described for Partial-Thickness and Full-Thickness Ulcers (excluding exposure of tendon, capsule, muscle, or bone).

Product
Hydrogels sheet (low exudate)

Frequency of Use
Once to twice daily

Procedure
- Same as described for Partial-Thickness and Full-Thickness Ulcers (excluding exposure of tendon, capsule, muscle, or bone).

Product
Moist gauze

Frequency of Use
Three times daily (must be kept moist)

Procedure
- Same as described for Partial-Thickness and Full-Thickness Ulcers (excluding exposure of tendon, capsule, muscle, or bone).

Product
Calcium alginates or hydrofibers (high exudate)

Frequency of Use
Once to twice daily

Procedure
- Same as described for Partial-Thickness and Full-Thickness Ulcers (excluding exposure of tendon, capsule, muscle, or bone).

Compression modalities vary in the amount of stretch and elasticity, both intrinsically and extrinsically, in the manner in which they are applied. Correct application is extremely important to product effectiveness. Considerations include:

- patient's daily activities
- patient's tolerance of compression modality
- number of dressing changes required per week
- cost-effectiveness
- grade of compression required
- ability to apply device (patient's and clinician's)
- wound status.

Note: Three- and four-layered wraps provide additional compression with each layer. Caution must be taken to appropriately apply each layer.

Table 9.1

Compression Modalities

Compression Modality	Advantages	Disadvantages
Stockings	Maintain desired compression Washable/reusable May be used on limbs with or without ulcers	May be expensive Often difficult to apply Should not be used with arterial disease, severe infection, weeping dermatitis, or friable tissue Do not absorb exudate Do not address skin and wound problems
Elastic wraps	Easy to apply Inexpensive Readily available	Should not be used with arterial disease, severe infection, weep-

Table 9.1 *(continued)*

Compression Modality	Advantages	Disadvantages
Elastic wraps *(continued)*		ing dermatitis, or friable tissue
		Difficult to keep in place
		May result in uneven compression
		Should not be used when severe inflammation is present
		Do not absorb exudate
		Do not address skin and wound problems
		Lose elasticity quickly
Elastic wraps (adherent with incorporated dressing)	Easy to apply	More expensive than conventional wraps
	Stay in place well	
	Help to prevent skin desiccation	Should not be used with arterial disease or infection
	Absorb some exudate	
		May damage fragile tissue
	May be therapeutic for dehydrated and damaged skin	May be applied incorrectly
		Cannot be worn bathing; limit daily hygiene
		Not to be used over weeping dermatitis or large ulcerations without additional dressings

Table 9.1 *(continued)*

Compression Modality	Advantages	Disadvantages
Three- and four-layered wraps	Easy to apply Apply high levels of pressure Nonmedicated Hypoallergenic Stay in place well Absorb some exudate Maintain pressure for up to 1 week	May be applied incorrectly Limit hygiene, bathing Should not be used with arterial disease or infection
Medicated wraps (non-adhesive) Unna's boot	Patient cannot disturb wound Moderate to low cost Maintain high level of compression during first 72 hours	Should not be used with arterial disease, severe infection, friable tissue Absorb limited exudate Cannot be worn bathing; limit daily hygiene May excessively dry, adhere to, and damage underlying skin Must be applied by experienced individual Aggravate problem when incorrectly applied Often uncomfortable to wear May lose compression benefits after 72 hours

Table 9.1 *(continued)*

Compression Modality	Advantages	Disadvantages
Pneumatic compression devices	Easy to use Predetermined levels of pressure applied Require minimal instruction in use Address underlying pathology	Sleeve may be difficult to apply Avoid with infection, heart failure, and severe arterial disease Do not eliminate need for compression stockings No clear-cut guidelines for amount of time pump should be used each day/week
Foot pumps	Easy to use Comfortable Require minimal instruction in use Self-adjusting; maintains target pressures automatically	May not be used with suspected preexisting deep vein thrombosis, heart failure, and infection Do not address the entire leg

Note: Stockings and pumps both provide reproducible and consistent pressure.

Dressing Materials

Wound dressings provide an optimal environment for wound repair, but they do not address the problem of increased venous return. They should be used to promote reepithelialization and granulation when the underlying pathophysiology has been treated.

Infected Ulcers

Occlusive compression dressings, bandages, wraps, and pneumatic sequential compression devices should not be used in the presence of clinical signs of infection or cellulitis.

Prevention

Venous ulcers may recur within days of healing if the venous disease is neglected after wound closure. Wound closure does not signify resolution of the patient's primary vascular problem. Continued use of compression therapy (particularly stockings and pneumatic compression devices) is crucial for ulcer prophylaxis.

Arterial Disease

Most prolonged compression is not recommended in the presence of severe arterial disease or an ankle-brachial index < 0.8. Clinicians should evaluate each patient on an individual basis.

Venous Ulcers Treatment Algorithm

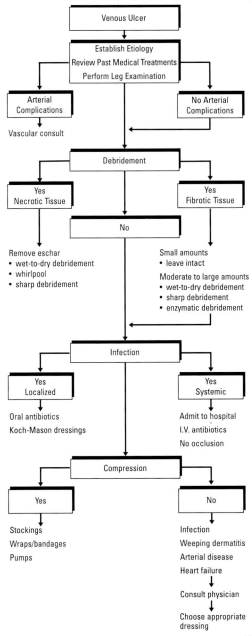

Venous Ulcer

Establish Etiology
Review Past Medical Treatments
Perform Leg Examination

Arterial
Complications

Vascular consult

No Arterial
Complications

Debridement

Yes
Necrotic Tissue

No

Yes
Fibrotic Tissue

Remove eschar
• wet-to-dry debridement
• whirlpool
• sharp debridement

Small amounts
• leave intact

Moderate to large amounts
• wet-to-dry debridement
• sharp debridement
• enzymatic debridement

Infection

Yes
Localized

Yes
Systemic

Oral antibiotics
Koch-Mason dressings

Admit to hospital
I.V. antibiotics
No occlusion

Compression

Yes

No

Stockings
Wraps/bandages
Pumps

Infection
Weeping dermatitis
Arterial disease
Heart failure

Consult physician

Choose appropriate
dressing

Diabetic Ulcers

The high morbidity and mortality associated with diabetic ulcers is attributed to the pathophysiology of the disease and inadequate knowledge of treatment principles for these ulcers.

Pathophysiology

Neuropathy and vascular disease are two major factors contributing to ulcer formation. Neuropathy generally affects the motor, sensory, and autonomic peripheral nerves of the leg, commonly presenting as a "stocking glove" paresthesia of the foot. Loss of feeling in the diabetic foot results in absence of sensitivity to pain, temperature, and pressure. When trauma occurs, the patient is unaware of tissue damage, inflammation, and infection until an ulcer becomes evident.

Many plantar ulcers result from pressure points, particularly calluses. As a result of altered skeletal biomechanics and atrophy of the underlying fat pad, reactive callus forms. Predominant areas of occurrence are submetatarsals, distal digits, medial fifth, second metatarsal head, and first metatarsophalangeal joint.

When seeking out the pulses on the foot, one should keep in mind the anatomic locations of the major vessels, although anomalies in this location are common. A portable Doppler device is preferred because it is an effective and inexpensive indicator of flow in larger vessels. Ideally, one would have access to a plethysmograph with digital attachments with a recorded readout.

Characteristics

- round, punched-out lesion with elevated rim
- periwound hyperkeratosis
- surrounding hyperkeratosis and anhidrosis
- eschar and necrotic debris in ulcer base uncommon (unless accompanied by vascular disease or infection)
- low to moderate drainage (unless infected)

Vascular disease found in diabetic patients is significantly different from nondiabetic patients. Diabetic vascular disease occurs at a younger age and is more accelerated. Occlusion usually involves the multisegmental small vessels. Signs of small vessel disease include:

- shiny skin
- digital redness
- dependent rubor
- loss of hair growth
- delayed superficial venous plexus filling time
- subcutaneous fat atrophy.

Evaluation

Patient evaluation includes:

- diabetic status
- nutritional status
- vascular status of affected extremity
- neurologic status
- ulcer status
- footwear.

Ulcer evaluation includes:

- size
- precise anatomical location
- stage of ulcer (some practitioners use the Wagner scale, which incorporates the level of infection of a wound)
- appearance of ulcer base
- description of amount and type of exudate
- periwound appearance
- exploration for sinus tracts, fistulas, and bone exposure.

Table 9.2

Wagner Ulcer Grade Classification	
Grade 0	• Preulcerative lesion • Healed ulcers • Presence of bony deformity
Grade 1	• Superficial ulcer without subcutaneous tissue involvement

Table 9.2 *(continued)*

Grade 2	• Penetration through the subcutaneous tissue (may expose bone, tendon, ligament, or joint capsule)
Grade 3	• Osteitis, abscess, or osteomyelitis
Grade 4	• Gangrene of digit
Grade 5	• Gangrene of the foot requiring disarticulation

Wagner FW, Jr. A classification and treatment program for diabetic, neuropathic, and dysvascular foot problems. AAOS Instruct Course Lect 1979;27:143.

Treatment

Preulceration

Discoloration of skin.

- Debride callus.
- Use accommodative devices such as foam, felt, and special shoes to offload or protect potential sites.
- Instruct patients on :
  - daily inspection of feet
  - foot hygiene
  - selection of proper footwear
  - discontinuance of "self-debridement" and the use of over-the-counter foot medications
  - education
  - continued medical care.

Partial-Thickness and Full-Thickness

Excluding exposure of tendon, capsule, muscle, or bone.

- Relieve pressure by using accommodative devices. Also, restrict patient to partial- or non-weight-bearing activities, when possible, by use of crutches.
- Debride callus.
- Prevent infection.
- Apply contact casting if the ulcer is resistant to other treatment. This cast should be applied only by an experienced individual.
- Apply appropriate dressings according to the package insert.

- Instruct patients on:
  - daily inspection of feet
  - foot hygiene
  - selection of proper footwear
  - discontinuance of "self-debridement" and the use of over-the-counter foot medications.

Product

Moist gauze

Frequency of Use

Two to three times per day.

Procedure

- Debride area of all necrotic tissue.
- Clean with normal saline or wound cleanser.
- Apply moist gauze and secure with dry gauze or covering.

Product

Hydrogels

Frequency of Use

Once to twice per day.

Procedure

- Debride area of all necrotic tissue.
- Clean with saline or wound cleanser.
- Apply hydrogel according to package insert.
- Cover with gauze or semipermeable foam wafer.

Note: Avoid using hydrogels and other moisture-retaining dressings with infected wounds unless indicated on package insert.

Product

Semipermeable foam wafer

Frequency of Use

Once per day (more frequently if heavily exudating).

Procedure

- Debride area of all necrotic tissue.
- Clean with normal saline or wound cleanser.
- Apply semipermeable foam wafer according to package insert and secure.

Product

Calcium alginates

Frequency of Use

Once per day (more frequently if heavily exudating).

Procedure

- Debride area of all necrotic tissue.
- Clean with normal saline or wound cleanser.
- Apply according to package insert.

Note: Totally occlusive dressings and products that hold high amounts of exudate on the wound surface should be avoided on diabetic patients. Newer occlusive technologies may allow a dressing to wick excess esudate away from the wound surface and retain it under pressure. Read package inserts carefully and use with extreme caution. Excessive moisture may promote maceration and decreased tissue tensile strength. Continued pressure and/or shear will produce greater tissue damage in the presence of maceration and decreased tissue tensile strength. Decreased cellular immune response may affect ability to reduce bacterial colorization. Bacterial proliferation may increase in the presence of excess moisture.

Full-Thickness

With exposure of tendon, capsule, muscle, or bone. Avoid adhesive coverings.

- Relieve pressure by using accommodative devices. Also, restrict patient to partial- or non-weight-bearing activities, when possible, by use of crutches.
- Debride callus and all necrotic tissue from wound.
- Prevent infection. Use sterile dressings daily.
- Rule out osteomyelitis
- Apply contact casting if the ulcer is resistant to other treatment and no osteomyelitis is present.
- Obtain surgical consult as needed.
- Apply appropriate dressings: moist gauze, hydrogels, and semipermeable foam wafers may be used as described on the preceding pages. Caution must be taken to rule out osteomyelitis or other infection.

- Instruct patients on:
  - daily inspection of feet
  - foot hygiene
  - selection of proper footwear
  - discontinuance of "self-debridement" and the use of over-the-counter foot medications.

Pressure Relief

Ideally, pressure relief for a foot ulcer means restriction to complete non-weight-bearing activities, and bedrest, if necessary. In an ambulatory patient, footwear should be modified to relieve pressure on the ulcer. Felt or high-density foam inserts, moldable Plastozote or other soft insoles, soft-soled healing shoes, or modified postoperative shoes may be of benefit. Use of crutches decreases further trauma to the ulcer. When patient compliance with bedrest and pressure relief is poor, contact casting, which redistributes pressure, is indicated.

Plantar Ulcers

Common locations of plantar ulcers on diabetic patients include:
- submetatarsals
- distal digits
- medial fifth
- second metatarsal head
- first metatarsophalangeal joint.

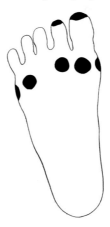

Debridement

Most diabetic ulcers are surrounded by a thick rim of keratinized tissue. Untreated, this will impede healing. Surgical debridement should extend through the callus and expose underlying pink viable tissue. All necrotic tissue needs to be debrided from the wound.

Sharp debridement is usually the most effective and efficient form of debridement. However, it should be done by an experienced individual. Eschar and fibrotic debris may be removed by enzymatic debriding agents (when minimal debris is present) or dressings described. Hydrotherapy (whirlpool) is used to soften and loosen eschar and debris, but it is not recommended.

Dressing Materials

Most diabetic ulcers are on a weight-bearing surface, making it difficult for hydrocolloids, hydrogel sheets, and thin film dressings to stay in place. They may be used on non-weight-bearing, low-exudating partial-thickness and some full-thickness ulcers. Silver sulfadiazine and gauze may be effective in reducing bacterial colonization on all low-exudate diabetic ulcers on both weight-bearing and non-weight-bearing surfaces. Silver sulfadiazine should be limited to 2 weeks maximum use. When applying silver sulfadiazine, place only a thin layer over the wound surface after the wound has been debrided and cleaned. Dressing should be changed every 24 hours.

Contact Casting

Contact casting is a specific type of below-the-knee cast that limits excessive foot motion and redistributes the body's weight over the entire foot. Patient compliance is improved because ambulation is permitted. Casts must be heavily padded over all bony prominences to prevent further tissue injury. Casts must be changed weekly and the ulcer evaluated for signs of infection. Appropriate training from individuals experienced with this technique is mandatory prior to applying contact casts. These casts are different from standard plaster casts. Casts should be removed when reepithelialization occurs.

Infected Ulcers

Bacterial infection is the most common complication of diabetic ulcers. Early diagnosis and treatment will reduce the threat of sepsis and limb loss. Hyperglycemia also must be controlled. Early detection of infected diabetic foot ulcers is difficult because symptoms of pain, erythema, and increased skin temperature may be masked by peripheral vascular disease and neuropathy. Prolonged hyperglycemia may be the first indication of infection.

Foot infections in diabetic patients are commonly polymicrobial and may involve aerobes and anaerobes. Prior to the administration of antibiotics, aerobic and anaerobic cultures should be obtained. Early superficial infections may be treated with oral antibiotics.

Treatment consists of local wound care and the use of systemic broad-spectrum antibiotics. Nonviable tissue must be debrided from the ulcer site.

Progressive cellulitis unresponsive to oral therapy, systemic signs of infection, abscess formation, and osteomyelitis require hospitalization and the use of I.V. antibiotics. Osteomyelitis may be difficult to differentiate from diabetic osteopathy and chronic inflammation with either X-ray or bone scan. A bone biopsy is the only definitive diagnosis for osteomyelitis. Surgical debridement of infected bone and a 6-week course of I.V. antibiotics may be required to eradicate osteomyelitis.

Tissue Replacements and Growth Factors

See Chapter 12, Wound Management: Past, Present, and Future.

Prevention

Once the ulcer is healed, patient education should include:
- instructions on daily foot care
- appropriate footwear
- daily inspection of feet and foot hygiene
- regularly scheduled visits to the health care professional.

Diabetic Ulcers Treatment Algorithm

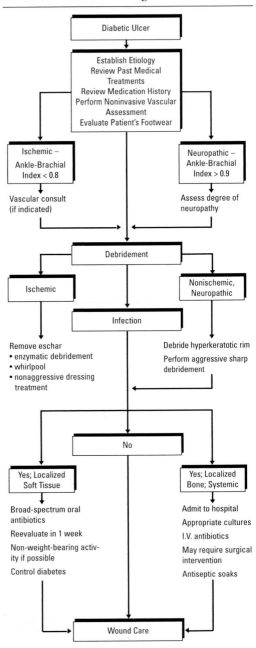

Diabetic Ulcer Wound Care Treatment Algorithm

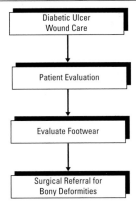

```
┌─────────────────────┐
│   Diabetic Ulcer    │
│    Wound Care       │
└─────────────────────┘
          │
          ▼
┌─────────────────────┐
│  Patient Evaluation │
└─────────────────────┘
          │
          ▼
┌─────────────────────┐
│  Evaluate Footwear  │
└─────────────────────┘
          │
          ▼
┌─────────────────────┐
│ Surgical Referral for│
│  Bony Deformities    │
└─────────────────────┘
```

Grade 0

- Padding and accommodative devices
- Debride callus
- Growth factor (rhPDGF-BB) when ABI > .45

Grade 1

- Follow Grade I protocol
- Topical silver sulfadiazine on highly contaminated wounds
- Nonocclusive dressing
- Evaluate weekly until healing
- Plantar surface – gauze dressing
- Dorsal surface – occlusive or nonocclusive dressing
- Growth factor (rhPDGF-BB) when ABI > .45

Grade 2

- Follow Grade I protocol
- R/O osteomyelitis (X-ray, scan, bone, biopsy)
- Non-weight-bearing
- Surgical consult
- Plantar surface – gauze dressing, amorphous hydrogel, alginate, or foam
- Dorsal surface – occlusive dressing
- Topical antimicrobial cream, ointment, or amorphous hydrogel
- Growth factor (rhPDGF-BB) when ABI > .45

Grade 3

- Follow Grade I protocol
- R/O osteomyelitis (X-ray, scan, bone, biopsy)
- Plantar surface – gauze dressing, amorphous hydrogel, alginate, or foam
- Dorsal surface – nonocclusive dressing
- Topical antimicrobial cream, ointment, or amorphous hydrogel

Grades 4 and 5

- Surgical consult and intervention

Arterial Ulcers

Arterial ulcers result from an inadequate blood supply. Any ulcer that fails to respond to conservative therapy should be examined closely for arterial insufficiency. Determining the ankle-brachial index will give an indication of a patient's ability to heal. One simply divides the ankle systolic pressure by the brachial systolic pressure. Patients with an index of less than 0.45 are not likely to heal (normal index = 1.0). (See page 75 for more information on ankle-brachial index values.)

Diabetic patients may have elevated indexes secondary to vessel calcification. Patients with these ulcers benefit most from revascularization procedures. When this is not possible, the goals of therapy should be to keep the patient comfortable and prevent wound deterioration.

Characteristics

- usually very painful
- pain often relieved by dependent leg position, aggravated by elevation
- minimal exudate
- commonly associated with dry necrotic eschar
- usually superficial
- present almost anywhere on leg; usually on dorsum of foot or on toes
- irregular shape and borders
- periwound tissue may appear blanched or purpuric
- periwound tissue often shiny and tight

Avoid using dressings that obscure signs of wound deterioration. Sharp debridement in the clinic setting should be avoided because further trauma to an area would result in an increase in wound size due to the lack of blood supply to the area.

The following algorithm is intended to provide basic recommendations for the treatment of arterial ulcers.

Arterial Ulcers Treatment Algorithm

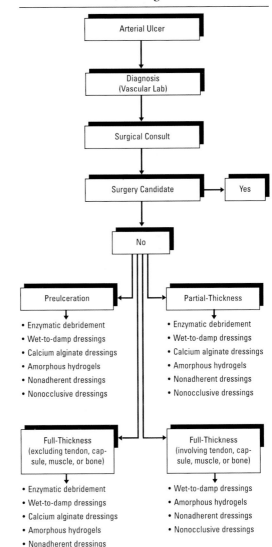

Arterial Ulcer

↓

Diagnosis
(Vascular Lab)

↓

Surgical Consult

↓

Surgery Candidate → Yes

↓

No

Preulceration

- Enzymatic debridement
- Wet-to-damp dressings
- Calcium alginate dressings
- Amorphous hydrogels
- Nonadherent dressings
- Nonocclusive dressings

Partial-Thickness

- Enzymatic debridement
- Wet-to-damp dressings
- Calcium alginate dressings
- Amorphous hydrogels
- Nonadherent dressings
- Nonocclusive dressings

Full-Thickness
(excluding tendon, capsule, muscle, or bone)

- Enzymatic debridement
- Wet-to-damp dressings
- Calcium alginate dressings
- Amorphous hydrogels
- Nonadherent dressings
- Nonocclusive dressings

Full-Thickness
(involving tendon, capsule, muscle, or bone)

- Wet-to-damp dressings
- Amorphous hydrogels
- Nonadherent dressings
- Nonocclusive dressings

Notes:

10

Diagnosis of Arterial Insufficiency

Arterial insufficiency or circulatory hypoperfusion most commonly results from atherosclerotic plaques that are large enough to narrow the arterial lumen. In general, a 50% reduction in arterial diameter on an arteriogram correlates with a 75% stenosis of a cross section. This produces resistance to flow and decreased downstream pressure.

The diagnosis of peripheral arterial disease hinges on a good history, physical examination, and prudent use of laboratory tests.

Table 10.1

Arterial Insufficiency Signs and Symptoms

- Arterial palpation (hardening of arteries and decreased pulses)
- Bruit
- Pallor of foot on elevation; rubor on dependency
- Temperature decrease in extremities
- Ischemic ulceration
- Necrosis and atrophy
- Integumentary changes
- Intermittent claudication
- Pain on elevation ("rest pain")

Clinical Findings

Signs

Physical examination is paramount in assessing the prevalence and severity of arterial disease.

Arterial palpation

Arteries often are hard and rubbery when atherosclerotic disease is present. Decreased amplitude of the pulse denotes a proximal stenosis. It is unusual for collateral flow to be sufficient to produce a pulse distal to an occluded artery.

Table 10.2

Grading of Pulses

4+	Normal
3+	Slightly reduced
2+	Markedly reduced
1+	Barely palpable
0	Absent

Bruit

Bruit indicates turbulent blood flow due to vibration of a blood vessel wall. It is heard loudest during systole and, with greater stenoses, may extend into diastole.

Pallor

Pallor of the foot on elevation of the extremity indicates advanced ischemia. Lesser degrees of elevation are necessary to produce pallor in patients with advanced lesions. The ischemia produced by elevation results in maximum cutaneous vasodilation. Thus, when the foot is returned to dependency, blood returns to the dilated bed producing an intense red, reactive hyperemia.

Rubor

Rubor is a cyanotic, purple discoloration of the foot on dependency. It appears because, with reduced inflow, blood in the capillary network is relatively stagnant and oxygen extraction is high. Hemoglobin becomes deoxygenated and the capillary blood has an increasing blue hue. Of note, the peripheral discoloration due to chronic congestion for venous insufficiency does not clear on elevation, which occurs in patients with arterial disease.

Temperature

With chronic ischemia, the temperature of the skin of the foot decreases. This is most important when there is a profound difference in temperature between the more and less ischemic extremities.

Ulceration

Ischemic ulcers usually are very painful and accompanied by ischemic rest pain of the foot. Typically, they occur on toes or at a site where trauma occurs. The margin of the ulcer is sharply demarcated or punched out, and the base is devoid of healthy granulation tissue. The surrounding skin is pale and mottled, and signs of chronic ischemia are invariably present.

Necrosis

Tissue necrosis first becomes apparent in the distal extremity or at an ulcer site. It stops at a line where the blood supply is sufficient to maintain viability. Dry gangrene appears first, but may become wet if secondary infection occurs.

Atrophy

Moderately severe degrees of chronic ischemia produce muscle atrophy and loss of strength in the ischemic zone. Frequently, there is associated decreased joint mobility of the foot as well. Subsequent changes in foot structure and gait increase the likelihood of developing ulcers.

Integumentary changes

Chronic ischemia commonly produces hair loss, thickened toenails, and shiny, scaly skin. Hence, a simple glance at a foot can help identify the presence or absence of serious arterial insufficiency.

Symptoms

Intermittent claudication

Intermittent claudication is pain or fatigue in muscles of the lower extremity produced by walking and relieved by rest. Typically, symptoms occur in the calf muscles, regardless of which arterial segment is involved. Claudication is distinguished from other pain in the extremities because some exertion is always required before it appears, it does not occur at rest, and it is relieved by cessation of walking. The two conditions that most commonly mimic claudication are osteoarthritis of the hip or knee and neurospinal compression due to narrowing of the lumbar neurospinal canal from osteophytosis (spinal stenosis).

Pain on elevation ("rest pain")

Ischemic rest pain is a grave symptom produced by far advanced arterial ischemia. It usually results in gangrene and amputation of the extremity if arterial reconstruction cannot be performed. In contrast to claudication, rest pain does not occur in a muscle group, but rather is described as a severe burning pain confined to the distal forefoot. Typically, it is aggravated by elevation of the extremity and relieved by dependency. Rest pain indicates an advanced stage of ischemia; it is classically preceded by claudication, but may occur de novo in patients whose walking is limited by other illnesses (e.g., angina pectoris).

Noninvasive Tests

A peripheral vascular testing laboratory should be equipped with a Doppler velocity detector, blood pressure cuffs of different sizes, a sphygmomanometer, and a motorized treadmill. In addition, a device to measure partial pressure of oxygen in tissues (transcutaneous $TCPO_2$) is useful. A device to measure toe pressures (e.g., plethysmograph, laser Doppler) is also important. Finally, a Duplex imaging system is not essential for the diagnosis of lower extremity vascular insufficiency, but it is crucial for other studies in the laboratory.

Table 10.3

Diagnostic Studies for Lower Extremity Vascular Insufficiency

- Segmental extremity pressure measurement
- Toe pressures
- Doppler waveform analysis
- Pulse Volume Recording
- $TCPO_2$
- Duplex scan
- Skin Perfusion Pressure

Segmental Pressure Measurement

A quick screening test for vascular insufficiency consists of measurement of resting systolic blood pressure at the brachial artery and the posterior tibial artery or the dorsal artery of the foot. The ankle-brachial index is determined by dividing the pressure obtained at the ankle by the brachial arterial pressure.

Table 10.4

Ankle-Brachial Index Values

>1.2	Suspect vessel wall calcification, stiffness (e.g., diabetes mellitus)
1.0 – 1.2	Normal
0.3 – 0.9	Claudication
0.0 – 0.3	Ischemic rest pain, nonhealing ulcers

In addition to the standard ankle-brachial index, segmental pressures can be obtained at various levels on the leg for localization of occlusive disease. Segmental pressures are performed as follows:

- Place patient in the supine position.
- Apply cuff to the high thigh, lower thigh, upper calf, and ankle.
- Use standard-sized (12 cm) adult cuffs for calf and ankle.
- Use larger (18 cm) cuffs for thigh pressures.
- Use highest brachial artery pressure for a denominator.
- Gradients of more than 20 mm Hg between sites are diagnostic of occlusive disease in the intervening segment.

Toe Pressure

Because of the common finding of inaccurately high ankle-brachial indexes in diabetic patients, measurement of toe pressure is particularly useful. In the normal person, there is a gradient of 20 to 30 mm Hg between the ankle and the toe; therefore, a correction must be made when toe pressures are being used. Healing of distal wounds can be expected when toe pressures are greater than 40 mm Hg. Healing rarely, if ever, occurs if toe pressures are less than 20 mm Hg. Pressures between 20 and 40 mm Hg are in a gray zone.

Doppler Waveform Analysis

Most commercial Doppler detectors provide an analog signal that is proportional to the velocity of blood in the vessel studied. The signal can be displayed on a screen or recorded for later analysis. The overall shape of the waveform reflects the status of the vessel proximal to the point studied. In the lower extremity, the normal velocity wave is triphasic, with reverse flow in early diastole. Proximal stenosis first eliminates the reverse flow, and with more severe lesions, there is bunting of the systolic upstroke and increasing flow during diastole.

Pulse Volume Recording

Blood entering a limb during systole causes an increase in the total volume in the extremity. During diastole, volume returns to normal. This phenomenon results in the pulse pressure oscillation seen with the sphygmomanometer while taking blood pressure. A variety of plethysmograph recorders have been devised using a mercury strain gauge, water displacement, and impedance. In the 1970s, the pulse volume recorder was developed to diagnose peripheral arterial disease. The diagnosis is based on the qualitative evaluation of the pulse volume waveform. Severe occlusive disease produces a flattened wave with a slow upstroke and downstroke. The absolute amplitude measurements are of limited value from patient to patient because substantial changes result from variations in cardiac output and vasomotor tone. However, comparison of amplitudes from one side to the other in the same patient may be useful for assessing unilateral disease. Like toe pressures, pulse volume recording is particularly useful when ankle-brachial index values do not seem accurate.

TCPO$_2$

Transcutaneous measurement of oxygen can be performed percutaneously using a special instrument. Determination of accurate TCPO$_2$ is difficult, however, and requires an experienced technician, patience, a warm room, and absence of vasoconstriction from other factors.

TCPO$_2$ should be measured on the dorsum, not the p . . tar aspect, of the foot. Ideally, a reference value is obtained at the chest. Analogous to absolute toe pressures, a TCPO$_2$ value of 40 mm Hg correlates with good healing, a TCPO$_2$ value below 20 mm Hg indicates poor or absent healing, and a TCPO$_2$ value between 20 and 40 mm Hg is in a gray zone.

Duplex Scan

A Duplex scan is used mostly for determination of occlusive disease in the carotid and intra-abdominal arteries. It also can document occlusive disease in the femoral artery. This technology is widely available in most vascular laboratories.

Skin Perfusion Pressure

Skin perfusion pressure is measured with a laser Doppler to provide a quantitative evaluation of small vessell disease. Measurement of skin perfusion pressure can be used to determine the presence of critical limb ischemia and aid in the determination of optimum clinical treatment for patients with diabetic foot ulcers. This test is not affected by edema, anemia, or medial calcification. The laser Doppler sensor has the precision needed for measurement of critically low blood pressures. This is a fast, reproducible, and convenient test.

Notes:

Chapter 11

MISCELLANEOUS
WOUNDS

11

Skin Tears

Treatment Objectives
- Protection
- Reepithelialization

Product
Transparent film dressing or thin hydrocolloid wafer

Frequency of Use
Every 3 to 5 days or if fluid leaks out.

Procedure
- Position patient off affected area.
- Gently clean affected area. Blot dry.
- Select a transparent film dressing or thin hydrocolloid wafer that allows at least a 2" margin of intact skin beyond the wound edge.
- Apply a skin sealant to all intact skin to be covered with dressing. Allow to dry until slick.
- Apply dressing, avoiding tension and skin wrinkling that would cause further damage.
- Write date of application and initials of applier directly on the dressing.

Product
Hydrocolloid or hydrogel wafer dressing

Frequency of Use
Every 3 to 7 days per package insert or if fluid leaks out.

Procedure
- Position patient off affected area.
- Use normal saline or a nonionic surfactant wound cleanser to remove wound debris and dressing material residue. Blot surrounding skin dry.
- Select a wafer that extends at least 2" beyond the wound area or cut a proper-sized piece from a larger wafer.
- Apply a skin sealant to periwound skin.

- Peel protective backing off wafer and center the dressing over the wound.
- Write date of application and initials of applier directly on the dressing.

Product

Creams/Ointments

Frequency of Use

Apply daily.

Procedure

- Position patient off affected area.
- Gently clean affected area. Blot dry.
- Apply small amount of cream/ointment and smooth into skin.

Extravasation Sites with Necrotic Tissue

Treatment Objectives

- Autolysis
- Granulation
- Reepithelialization

Product

Transparent film or thin transparent hydrocolloid wafer

Frequency of Use

Every 24 to 48 hours until necrotic tissue has been eliminated or if wound fluid leaks out. Then every 3 to 5 days to promote reepithelialization.

Procedure

- Gently clean affected area. Blot dry.
- Select a transparent thin dressing or thin hydrocolloid wafer that allows at least a 2" margin of intact skin beyond the wound edge.
- Apply a skin sealant to all intact skin to be covered with dressing. Allow to dry until slick.
- Apply dressing, avoiding tension and skin wrinkling that would cause further damage.
- Write date of application and initials of applier directly on the dressing.

Note: This procedure is useful for high-risk neonates for whom surgery is contraindicated.

Treatment Objectives
- Debridement
- Granulation
- Reepithelialization

Product
Amorphous hydrogel dressing (for nonexudating wounds only)

Frequency of Use
Every 24 hours.

Procedure
- Position patient off affected area.
- Use normal saline or a nonionic surfactant wound cleanser to remove wound debris and dressing material residue.
- Blot surrounding skin dry.
- Apply skin sealant to periwound skin. Allow to dry until slick.
- Lightly coat the wound bed with the amorphous hydrogel. If there is a deep cavity, lightly pack with an impregnated hydrogel gauze or hydrofiber dressing.
- Cover with a nonadherent dressing or a transparent film dressing.
- Secure with hypoallergenic tape, if needed.

Note: Use stretch gauze wrap or self-adhesive fabric tape to secure dressing over bony prominences. Montgomery straps may be used to secure dressing to avoid frequent tape removal.

Product
Calcium alginate or hydrofiber (exudating wounds only)

Frequency of Use
Every 24 to 72 hours depending on amount of wound exudate. Discontinue when wound drainage ceases.

Procedure
- Position patient off affected area.
- Use normal saline or a nonionic surfactant wound

cleanser to remove wound debris and dressing
material residue.

- Blot surrounding skin dry.
- Apply skin sealant to periwound skin. Allow to dry
  until slick.
- Select a calcium alginate or hydrofiber dressing
  the size of the wound or cut a piece to fit from a
  larger dressing.
- Place in wound bed.
- Cover with a nonadherent dressing, absorbent
  gauze, nonwoven pad, transparent film dressing,
  or semipermeable foam dressing.
- Secure cover dressing with hypoallergenic tape, if
  needed.

*Note: Use stretch gauze wrap or self-adhesive fabric
tape to secure dressing over bony prominences.
Montgomery straps may be used to secure dressing to
avoid frequent tape removal. A brownish green viscous
residue may appear in the wound bed or in soiled
dressings. This probably is a dressing by-product.
Evaluate the wound after thorough, gentle irrigation.*

Gastrointestinal/Genitourinary Fistulas

Treatment Objectives
- Evacuate
- Collect
- Protect surrounding skin

Product
Closed-suction wound drainage

Frequency of Use
Every 5 to 7 days or if surgeon desires to examine wound.
Change if wound drainage leaks out of dressing.

Procedure
- Position patient off affected area.
- Use normal saline or a nonionic surfactant wound
  cleanser to remove needle debris.
- Open completely one 2x2 gauze square. Lay
  across the wound bed. (For cutaneous fistula,
  encircle the opening with a pectin-based barrier or

hydrocolloid wafer dressing to form a trough for the fenestrated drain. No need for 2x2 gauze lining.)

- Place Jackson Pratt drain in the wound bed, not in the fistula tract.
- Open two 4x4 gauze squares. Saturate with normal saline. Fluff into wound to completely cover the drain and fill the defect to skin level.
- Apply skin sealant to all intact skin that will be covered by transparent film dressing. Allow to dry until slick.
- Cut transparent film dressing or select size to allow at least 1" of intact skin beyond wound edges. Place transparent film dressing over packed wound. Crimp transparent film dressing around the tube against the skin.
- Reinforce tube exit site with waterproof tape to ensure an airtight seal.
- Connect the end of the drain to the wall suction tubing.
- Turn on continuous suction to the upper range of the low setting, approximately 60 to 80 mm Hg, and observe the wound site. The dressing should contract noticeably. If it does not, you do not have a closed system and wound drainage will override it.

Note: A small "Christmas tree" connector is ideal to connect the end of the drain to wall suction tubing if end of fenestrated drain does not fit snugly into suction canister tubing. Do not attempt to use bulb of Jackson Pratt system. If fistula effluent is thick, disconnect fenestrated tubing from canister tubing and gently irrigate with normal saline until patent, then reconnect. Fenestrated drain may be washed and reused at dressing changes.

Product
Large wound drainage collector

Procedure
Apply according to manufacturer's instructions.

Radiation Burns

Treatment Objectives
- Pain control
- Odor control
- Drainage containment

Pain Control

- Cover dry or lightly draining wounds with hydrogel wafer and change daily. Or apply small amount of amorphous hydrogel three times daily. Cover with nonadherent dressing and change daily.
- Use soft net wraps or stretch mesh briefs, or tailor cotton jersey undershirts or underpants to hold dressings in place.
- Do not use dressings that adhere to the wound or surrounding radiation-damaged skin.
- Do not use tape on damaged irradiated skin or to secure dressings that require frequent removal and reapplication.

Odor Control

- Use activated charcoal dressings or gauze soaked with chlorophyllin copper complex solution.
- Select a deodorizing spray that does not mask odor with a pungent scent and that is not harmful to skin. Spray directly on the outer dressing as needed.
- Use compresses soaked in 1% metronidazole solution on lesion 20 minutes twice a day, followed by a moist or nonadherent dressing.
- Use 0.75% metronidazole gel in the wound according to the package insert.

Drainage Containment

- Use a dressing designed for lightly draining wounds.
- Pouch a profusely draining wound with an ostomy type pouch or large wound drainage collector.
- Use closed suction wound drainage (see Gastro-intestinal/Genitourinary Fistulas, pages 82 and 83).

Chapter 12

WOUND MANAGEMENT: PAST, PRESENT, AND FUTURE

12

Past

Wine, turpentine, feathers, sugar, and combinations such as bismuth and bourbon, clay and spittle, povidone-iodine and sugar, and milk of magnesia and merbromin are all substances that have been applied to pressure ulcers and other lesions. None has proven efficacy based on sound scientific studies.

Current and Future

Dressings that maintain a moist wound environment are recommended. Transparent adhesive dressings, foams, hydrocolloid and hydrogel dressings, and calcium alginates have distinct advantages over plain or impregnated gauze. Clinicians should evaluate product information and published studies before making treatment decisions.

Biologic Materials: Tissue Substitutes

Biologic materials, designed to act as temporary or permanent tissue substitutes, are being researched. Tissue substitutes contain human cells that may secrete growth factors and matrix proteins important to the wound repair process. Valid studies are needed to determine the benefits of biologic materials, i.e., tissue substitutes over other materials such as alginates, foams, and hydrocolloids. The treatment of acute and chronic wounds may yet be revolutionized by the introduction of tissue engineering — the science of growing living human tissue equivalents.

Cultured keratinocytes have been studied for over a decade. These materials are autologous, are most useful on clean partial-thickness wounds, and must be reapplied to the same patient from which the cells were obtained. Their use on the chronic wound is limited by cost, availability, and autologous application. The most recently studied products fall into two categories, a bilayered skin equivalent and human dermal replacement.

Bilayered Skin Equivalent

The only extensively researched bilayered skin equivalent (Apligraf, Organogenesis Inc., Canton, MA) is an allogenic skin equivalent that has been tested extensively in controlled trials in venous ulcers and dermatologic surgery. This device contains a dermal matrix with viable fibroblasts in a collagen lattice and an epidermis made up of a cornified differentiated layer of keratinocytes. The purpose of this device is to assist with the reestablishment of new skin tissue through stimulation of the wound bed by its cellular components. It has some features and applications that are sometimes compared to a skin graft. This bilayered skin equivalent has been studied in clinical trials and found to be effective in promoting wound healing in venous ulcers, particularly recalcitrant venous ulcers of long duration. The product is not designed to address the underlying venous disease. Apligraf is currently FDA approved for use on venous ulcers.

Human Dermal Replacement

Currently, a tissue-engineered human dermal replacement is being studied on diabetic foot ulcers. This product has not yet been approved for use on diabetic foot ulcers in the United States. It is a three-dimensional cultivation of human diploid fibroblast cells on a polymer scaffold. The fibroblasts are living and are metabolically active following implantation into the wound bed. Fibroblasts are known to secrete a combination of growth factors and matrix proteins, which contribute to tissue regeneration and wound healing. This device has been designed to replace the dermal layer of skin and provide the stimulus for a normal wound healing process.

The success of cultured-cell technology in the clinical setting is dependent on a number of factors, including:

- wound condition
- patient's general medical status
- patient's ambulatory status

- patient compliance
- wound preparation prior to application.

Future applications of tissue engineering may provide products that may change and revolutionize wound treatment.

Electrical Stimulation

Numerous articles are available on the benefits of electrical stimulation for bone healing. The role of electrical stimulation in wound repair has not been clearly defined. Although many articles support its use and claim significant gains in expediting wound repair, no consistently defined regimen that can be reliably duplicated by other investigators exists. More research is indicated to determine the type and means of application that is most beneficial to chronic wounds. Electrical stimulation should be considered as adjunctive treatment to nonresponsive wounds.

Growth Factors

Growth factors are polypeptide molecules whose activities affect the wound repair process, including cell metabolism, differentiation, and growth. They may stimulate different functions including angiogenesis, enzyme production, cell migration, chemotaxis, and cellular proliferation. Growth factors, also described as cytokines, interleukins, and colony-stimulating factors, are named according to their function, their cell of origin, or the target cell toward which their action is directed. The presence or absence of growth factors may significantly influence the wound closure process.

Several growth factors believed to affect wound closure have been studied. Autologous growth factors may be isolated from a patient's blood and applied to their chronic wound. Genetic recombinant growth factors are currently being researched. Prospective, randomized double-blind trials are needed to provide supporting scientific evidence for their role and need in chronic wounds. Clinically studied growth factors include transforming growth factor beta, fibroblast growth factor, platelet-derived growth factor, and epidermal growth factor.

Currently, the only growth factor approved by the Food and Drug Administration is becaplermin (REGRANEX Gel 0.01%, Ortho McNeil Pharmaceutical, NJ). This trade drug is the only growth factor (rhPDGF-BB) to demonstrate clinical efficacy and to be approved for the treatment of diabetic neuropathic foot ulcers. Clinical trials also have shown rhPDGF-BB to be safe and well tolerated. Indications for other use, including venous and pressure ulcers, are anticipated in the near future. This growth factor stimulates the migration and proliferation of many cell types involved in wound repair. Fibroblasts also express receptors for rhPDGF-BB and may be responsive to this growth factor. Additional functions of rhPDGF-BB include chemotaxis for mesenchymal-derived cells and stimulation of fibroblast proliferation, osteoblasts, and smooth-muscle cells. The product is indicated to promote closure of chronic lower extremity diabetic neuropathic foot ulcers. As with all products, it should be used as indicated and with standard administration of good adjunctive wound care.

Extensive research still is needed to determine the effect of other growth factors and their influence on nonhealing wounds. It is still unknown when particular growth factors are deficient in the nonhealing wound, how much is needed, when it is needed, how much should be applied, and what the precise physiologic response will be. Costs and benefits need to be carefully reviewed by the clinician.

Hyperbaric Oxygen Therapy

Hyperbaric oxygen therapy has been advocated for selected nonhealing wounds and anaerobic wound infections. Patients are treated in multiplace or monoplace chambers for several hours once or twice daily for several days depending on the problem. Topical oxygen chambers for extremities deliver oxygen to the wound site but are not hyperbaric. Their value in chronic wounds is questionable and the cost of treatment is expensive.

Interactive and Active Dressings

Dressings that interact with the wound's environment are emerging. These include calcium alginates and certain hydrocolloid and hydrogel wafer dressings that can deliver substances to the wound to stimulate healing.

Normothermic Dressing/Device

The normothermic dressing/device (Warm–Up Active Wound Therapy, Augustine Medical, Inc., Eden Prarie, MN) optimizes local wound environment by providing levels of heat to a wound. The device is described as a "mini-greenhouse," consisting of a foam collar applied to the periwound skin. A transparent film covers the top of the collar and is raised above the level of the wound. An infrared warming card is inserted into a pocket built into the film covering. When turned on, the warming card raises the temperature inside the dressing to 38°C, providing an environment favorable to neutrophil function and cellular metabolism. Pilot studies of about 40 patients have indicated a significant improvement in wound healing over standard wound care.

Vacuum Assisted Closure

Vacuum assisted closure (V.A.C., KCI, San Antonio, TX) consists of a medical grade open-cell foam dressing, which is placed into the wound bed and covered with an occlusive film dressing. A negative pressure ("vacuum") of 125 mm Hg is applied to the dressing. In two recently published studies, wounds treated with this method closed more quickly than similar wounds treated with conventional nonsurgical treatments. Vacuum assisted closure has been used successfully in the treatment of chronic, nonhealing wounds such as pressure ulcers, venous ulcers, dehiscence, and burns.

Ultrasound

Ultrasound is a form of physical therapy used for the treatment of soft-tissue trauma, hematosis and inflammation, and induration. Therapeutic benefits are well documented. Well-designed, controlled randomized clinical trials are needed to determine its place in wound treatment.

Currently, purported benefits of ultrasound include:
- increased oxygen transport
- decreased pain
- expedited wound closure
- increased angiogenesis
- decreased edema.

Whirlpool

Use warm isotonic solution for optimal patient comfort and wound response (6 pounds salt for 75 gallons, 21 pounds salt for 270 gallons and 33 pounds salt for 425 gallons). Use whirlpool to soften necrotic tissue prior to debridement. Discontinue when wound is clean or does not require immediate debridement. Avoid whirlpool on diabetic patients. Whirlpool is usually not indicated for most wounds. It is recommended in cases in which it will significantly assist with debridement.

Support Surface Properties

Special support surfaces play a key role in the prevention and treatment of pressure ulcers. Specialty surfaces have been available for decades. However, the last 5 years have been a time of explosive growth and marketing of these surfaces. In spite of the rapid growth of this market, special support surfaces are a source of misunderstanding, misuse, misinformation, and frustration. When selecting a support surface, the properties of these devices should be taken into consideration and matched to the needs of the patient and staff. These properties include interface pressure, friction and shear characteristics, moisture vapor transmission rate, thermal insulation properties, indentation load deflection, density, ease of use, safety, and patient comfort.

Interface Pressure Measurement

Probably the most commonly used means to compare support surfaces is the interface pressure measurement. Interface pressure is a measure of the force the support surface applies to the tissue it is supporting. The most common areas where interface pressures are measured are between the support surface and the bony prominences, such as trochanters, sacrum, coccyx, heels, and occiput. With the widespread use of this tool, new terminology was developed to make the measurements more useful. Thus, the terms *pressure relief* and *pressure reduction* were introduced. Pressure relief was defined as pressure below 25 to 32 mm Hg. Pressure reduction was defined as the reduction of interface pressures to 26 to 32 mm Hg, but not consistently. Although somewhat useful in evaluating support surfaces, interface pressures are not the precise standard needed as a basis for major decisions on patient care and cost control. The problem arises from several issues associated with interface pressures.

One problem is the fact that the standard of 32 mm Hg, as the capillary closing pressure, was measured in healthy young males. It is now known that interface pressures in elderly patients can be as low as 12 mm Hg. Another problem with using interface pressures as the sole criterion in evaluating support surfaces is the fact that they are not highly repeatable when measured by different persons, different devices, and even the same person and device on different days. The terms *pressure relief* and *pressure reduction* have been rendered useless by the marketing tactics of manufacturers. Although interface pressures are a reasonable place to start in evaluating a product, the decision to use a product should not be based solely on this parameter.

Friction

Friction is another valuable measure of a support surface's ability to prevent and treat skin breakdown. Friction can be described as the amount of resistance generated between two objects as they are moved in opposite directions — in other words, how much the two surfaces want to stick together.

Friction is commonly described as the coefficient of friction. The higher the coefficient, the higher the frictional drag. The higher the frictional drag, the more likely the patient's skin can be denuded during repositioning. A high coefficient of friction also means that shear forces are high. Shear occurs when two surfaces are being moved in opposite directions and the friction forces do not allow the surfaces to slide freely across each other. Shear commonly occurs when patients are moved up in bed without being completely lifted off the surface of the bed. As the patient is moved up in bed, the skin adheres to the sheet and mattress. The blood vessels supplying the skin may be angulated or kinked and blood flow can be disrupted. Friction and shear forces increase as moisture on the surfaces increases. This is a good reason to evaluate the moisture vapor transmission rate of the support surface under consideration.

Moisture Vapor Transmission Rate

Moisture vapor transmission rate is the measure of a fabric's ability to move moisture through the fabric from one side to the other side or away from the patient's skin through the fabric. The rate of moisture vapor transmission is measured in milliliters of water per square meter per 24 hours ($ml/m^2/24$ hour). It has been determined that in order to prevent overhydration of the skin, a transmission rate of at least 300 $ml/m^2/24$ hour is needed. There are several methods used to measure this rate. When comparing transmission rate between two fabrics, make sure to compare values obtained with the same method.

Thermal Insulation Properties

Another variable to consider is the thermal insulation properties of the support surface. Thermal insulation is an important characteristic for two reasons. One, if the device has poor thermal properties, then the patient may have to expend more energy trying to maintain a comfortable temperature. Two, if the device has a heating system, then thermal properties may not be a critical factor in selecting a product. If the product has a high thermal insulation value, then the patient may not be able to eliminate excess heat. The patient may increase sensible and insensible water losses in order to maintain a normal temperature. The increase in moisture against the skin will increase friction and shear. Overhydrated skin cells are not a good barrier to bacteria.

Indentation Load Deflection

If the product being evaluated is made of foam, the following properties need to be taken into consideration: indentation load deflection, support factor, and density. Indentation load deflection is a measurement of load-bearing capacity or firmness. It is also known as indentation force deflection, and the terms are interchangeable. Indentation load deflection is measured with specific equipment, according to the procedure described in the American Society for Testing and Materials 3574 test. To determine 25% deflection, a sample of foam is compressed 25% so that its new height is 75% of the original height. The amount of force required to achieve this 25% compression is the 25% indentation load deflection. The 25% deflection should be between 25 and 35 lb.

Support Factor

Another commonly measured indentation load deflection is the 65% deflection. This is the force required to compress the sample of foam to 35% of its original height. Dividing the 65% deflection by the 25% deflection gives the relationship of support to comfort known as the support factor. Names for this measurement are the sag factor, hardness ratio, or comfort factor. The higher the number, the greater the difference between the surface firmness and the deep-down support. The support factor is the best means of measuring comfort for comparison. Higher support factors indicate desirable surface softness and firm inner support.

Density

Density is the weight of a cubic foot of foam. Weight of foam can vary according to the amount of urethane used in the manufacturing process or the addition of other chemicals. Density is measured in pounds per cubic foot. Density is independent of firmness and is considered to be a good indicator of the overall quality of the foam. Foam with a density of 1.8 lb/cu ft or higher is less likely to bottom out during clinical use and is less likely to fatigue, which reduces effectiveness and life of the foam.

Ease of Use

The next property to be examined is ease of use. If a product is labor-intensive and has marginal superiority over similar devices, is it cost-effective from a time management perspective? Does the product have superior outcome studies that would offset the increase in time required to use the product correctly? Most differences between products can be adequately addressed with in-servicing provided by company representatives. It is important to have a vendor that provides in-servicing and routine servicing during the use of the product. Many companies provide educational programs discussing their products and issues that their products address. These companies may use other support services that can be accessed. Commonly, these extra services are part of contract negotiations.

Outside Testing

Special support surfaces must provide a safe environment for the patient and the staff. This means that the product should undergo testing by an outside agency such as Underwriters Laboratories. Specialized tests, regarding infection-control procedures for decontamination of the product, should be conducted by the manufacturer, but also should be replicated by another agency. Certain states have their own, more stringent requirements regarding product safety and performance. Most manufacturers will call your attention to possible safety concerns through warning labels attached to the product and discussion in the product literature. Examples of this would be a warning label that a product contains magnets, a product is made from latex, or that use of mattress overlays may increase the height of the patient surface and extended side rails are recommended.

The caregiver should always ask the question, what happens if the system fails? Is there a backup system built into the product? All systems are subject to failure, so how can you recognize failure in the product you are using? Does the product have an alarm? Does the product have enough margin of error that failure of the system will not result in catastrophic results for the patient? In the event of a system failure, the company needs to be notified and appropriate documentation needs to be initiated by the end user.

Support Surface Categories

There have been numerous attempts to categorize special support surfaces. They have been labeled as pressure relief or pressure reduction, framed or unframed, air flotation or air suspension, and so forth. What this means is that there is a great deal of confusion regarding support surfaces. In fact, there is so much confusion that several groups are currently trying to develop systems to categorize support surfaces. The system currently favored by one federal agency follows. It includes descriptions of alternating pressure pads, beds, mattress overlays, mattress replacements, and enhanced overlays and mattresses.

Alternating Pressure Pads

Alternating Pressure Pads	Recommended cell depth (pad and pump) should be not less than $2^{1}/_{2}$"

Beds

Air Fluidized Bed	Integrated system of support surface and bed frame. Air is circulated through silicone microspheres creating a fluid like state; also known as bead beds, sand beds, and high-air-loss beds.
Low-Air-Loss Bed	Integrated support system and bed frame. Interconnected air cells with a minimum depth of 5". The system allows for air to escape from the surface. This system has a dedicated power supply unit.
Low-Air-Loss Bed with Adjuvant Features	Integrated support system with bed frame. Interconnected air cells with a minimum depth of 5". The system allows for air to escape from the surface. The system has a dedicated power supply unit. These systems may provide other therapies (e.g., pulsation, percussion, kinetic).

Mattress Overlays

Air	Interconnected cells inflated with a pump. Recommended cell depth should not be less than 3".

Foam	For contoured foam, the base height and the height from the bottom of the foam to the start of the contour should not be less than 2". For the contoured foam, the overall height should not be less than $3\frac{1}{2}$". The density of the foam should be between 1.35 and 1.8 lb/cu ft. The 25% indentation load deflection should be between 25 and 35 lb. A waterproof cover that reduces shear and friction is recommended.
Gel	Recommended depth should not be less than 2".
Water	Recommended depth should not be less than 3".

Mattress Replacements

Air	Minimum recommended height is 5". A waterproof cover that reduces shear and friction is recommended. Should have at least a 2-year warranty.
Foam	Recommended minimum height of 5". Density should be between 1.35 and 1.8 lb/cu ft. The 25% indentation load deflection should be between 25 and 35 lb. A waterproof cover that reduces shear and friction is recommended. Should have at least a 2-year warranty.
Gel	Minimum recommended height is 5". A waterproof cover that reduces shear and friction is recommended. Should have at least a 2-year warranty.
Water	Minimum recommended height is 5". A waterproof cover that reduces shear and friction is recommended. Should have at least a 2-year warranty.

Alternating Pressure Mattress	Minimum recommended depth is 5". The configuration of the system's chambers allows for cyclical change of pressures in different chambers creating low- and high-pressure areas.
Low-Air-Loss Overlay	Overlay interconnected system of air cells with a minimum cell depth of 3". The system allows for air to escape from the surface.
Nonpowered Adjustable Zone Overlay	Must have at least three independent zones. The manifold system should provide constant force equalization within each section. Cover material should have a low coefficient of friction.
Low-Air-Loss Mattress	Interconnected air cells with a minimum depth of at least 5". The system allows air to escape from the surface. The system has a dedicated power supply unit.
Low-Air-Loss Mattress with Adjuvant Features	Interconnected air cells with a minimum depth of at least 5". The system allows for air to escape from the surface. The system has a dedicated power supply unit. These systems may provide other therapies (e.g., pulsation, percussion, kinetic).

Support Surface Manufacturers

Beginning on the next page is a list of support surface manufacturers with locations and phone numbers. This list is as accurate and comprehensive as possible at the date of publication. Each company represented here manufactures surfaces with varying properties. Match these properties to the needs of the patient and staff before making purchasing decisions.

American Health Systems, Inc.	Greenville, SC (864) 234-0496
Anatomic Concepts, Inc.	Corona, CA (800) 874-7237
Atlantis Medical Inc.	New Brunswick, NJ (800) 297-6060
B.G. Industries	Northridge, CA (800) 822-8288
Comfortex, Inc.	Winona, MN (800) 445-4007
Creative Bedding Technologies, Inc.	Elgin, IL (800) 526-2158
Crown Therapeutics, Inc.	Belleville, IL (800) 851-3449
Dermacare	Louisville, KY (800) 626-4550
EHOB, Incorporated	Indianapolis, IN (800) 966-3462
Gaymar Industries, Inc.	Orchard Park, NY (800) 828-7341
Grant Airmass Corporation (Dynacare)	Stamford, CT (800) 243-5237
Hermell Products, Inc.	Bloomfield, CT (800) 233-2342
Hill-Rom	Charleston, SC (800) 528-9593
Huntleigh Healthcare, Inc.	Manalapan, NJ (800) 223-1218
Integrated Therapy Products, Inc.	Jackson, MS (800) 748-7834
Invacare Corporation	Elyria, OH (800) 333-6900

James Consolidated, Inc.	Walnut Creek, CA (800) 884-3317
Jefferson Industries, Inc.	Lakewood, NJ (800) 257-5145
Ken McRight Supplies, Inc.	Tulsa, OK (918) 492-9657
Kinetic Concepts, Inc. (KCI)	San Antonio, TX (800) 531-5346
LifePlus Health Products	Thousand Oaks, CA (888) 449-4962
Lotus Health Care Products	Naugatuck, CT (800) 243-2362
Lumex Medical Products	Bayshore, NY (800) 645-5272
Mason Medical Products	Glendale, NY (800) 233-4454
Medifloat	Ormond Beach, FL (800) 678-9299
Med-I-Pant, Inc.	Champlain, NY (800) 361-4964
MEDIQ/FST	Pennsauken, NJ (800) 490-4744
Medline Industries, Inc.	Mundelein, IL (888) 701-SKIN
Mellen Air Manufacturing, Inc.	Long Beach, CA (800) 770-6264
Neuropedic	Clarks Summit, PA (800) 327-6759
Next Generaton Co., Inc.	Temecula, CA (800) 598-4303
Nova Health Systems, Inc.	Blackwood, NJ (800) 225-6682

Pegasus Airwave Inc.	Boca Raton, FL (800) 443-4325
Perry Baromedical	Riviera Beach, FL (800) 741-4376
Plexus Medical	San Dimas, CA (800) 690-6113
Recovercare, Inc.	Pennsauken, NJ (800) 579-2337
Regency Products International	Los Angeles, CA (800) 845-7931
ROHO, Inc.	Belleville, IL (800) 850-7646
Senior Technologies, Inc.	Lincoln, NE (800) 983-3287
SenTech Medical Systems	Ft. Lauderdale, FL (800) 474-4225
SleepNet Corporation	Manchester, NH (800) 742-3646
Span-America Medical Systems, Inc.	Greenville, SC (800) 888-6752
Spinal Technologies	Lakewood, NJ (800) 257-5145
Standard Textile Company, Inc.	Cincinnati, OH (800) 999-0400
Sundance Enterprises, Inc.	White Plains, NY (800) 942-0535
Sunrise Medical Continuing Care Group	Stevens Point, WI (800) 688-4083
Tempur-Medical, Inc.	Lexington, KY (800) 878-8889
Tetra Medical Supply Corp.	Niles, IL (800) 621-4041

Turnsoft Inc.	Huntersville, NC
	(800) 944-8876
Universal Hospital Services, Inc.	Bloomington, MN
	(800) 847-7368
Veritas Enterprises, Inc.	White Plains, NY
	(888) 765-6257
Zimmer, Inc.	Warsaw, IN
	(800) 613-6131

*Every effort has been made to include all manufacturers in this list. If manufacturers were omitted, it was not intentional. Reader recommendations for additions and deletions are encouraged. Any omission will be included in the next edition upon written notification of Springhouse Corporation. No endorsement of any product or manufacturer is intended.

Wound Care Products

Beginning on the next page are wound care products and
manufacturers arranged by category. Parentheses around
company names indicate companies from outside the
United States. This list is as accurate and comprehensive
as possible at the date of publication. Each product has
varying properties. Match these properties to the needs of
the patient and staff before making treatment decisions.

Antifungals

- treat jock itch, ringworm, and athletes foot

Examples:

Aloe Vesta Antifungal Ointment	ConvaTec, A Bristol-Myers Squibb Company
BAZA Cream Antifungal Barrier	Coloplast Corporation
Carrington Antifungal Cream with 2% Miconazole Nitrate	Carrington Laboratories Inc.
Critic-Aid Skin Paste	Coloplast Corporation
Ferni Clear Care Lotion	Ferno Ille
LOTRIMIN	Schering-Plough Healthcare Products, Inc.
Micro-Guard Cream	Coloplast Corporation
Mitrazol Cream	Healthpoint Medical
Mitrazol Powder	Healthpoint Medical
Triple Care Antifungal Cream Formula	Smith & Nephew, Inc.
Triple Care Antifungal Extra-Thick Formula	Smith & Nephew, Inc.
Vicatin	Advance/Ortho

Calcium Alginates

- highly absorbent (thick fibers absorb more exudate), interactive dressing
- convert into viscous hydrophilic gel after contact with exudate
- trapped fibers in wound are biodegradable
- enable autolysis of devitalized tissue

Examples:

3M Tegagen HI and HG Alginate Dressing	3M Health Care

Advanced Alginate	Hyperion Medical, Inc.
AlgiDERM Calcium Alginate Dressing	Bard Medical Division
AlgiSite Wound Dressing	Smith & Nephew, Inc.
Calcium Alginate	Gentell, Inc.
Calcium Alginate Membrane Pad Dressings	Ferris Manufacturing Corporation
Calcium Alginate Strip Dressings	Ferris Manufacturing Corporation
Calgicel	Glenwood
Carra-Sorb H Calcium Alginate Wound Dressing	Carrington Laboratories Inc.
CarraGinate Calcium Alginate Wound Dressing with Acemannan Hydrogel	Carrington Laboratories Inc.
Comfeel SeaSorb 16" Rope	Coloplast Corporation (Coloplast A/S)
Comfeel SeaSorb Dressing	Coloplast Corporation (Coloplast A/S)
CURADERM	Kendall Healthcare Products Company
CURASORB	Kendall Healthcare Products Company
Dermacea Alginate	Sherwood-Davis & Geck
DermAssist Calcium Alginate	AssisTec Medical, Inc.
DermaStat	Derma Sciences, Inc.
FyBron	B. Braun Medical Inc.
Kalginate	DeRoyal Wound Care
KALTOSTAT Dressing	ConvaTec, A Bristol-Myers Squibb Company
KALTOSTAT Fortex	ConvaTec, A Bristol-Myers Squibb Company

KALTOSTAT Rope	ConvaTec, A Bristol-Myers Squibb Company
Phyto Derma-Wound Gel	Aloe Life International
Restore CalciCare	Hollister Incorporated
SORBSAN	Dow Hickam Pharmaceuticals (Maersk) (Pharma-Plast, Ltd., Steriseal Division)

Charcoal Dressings

- absorb exudate
- reduce the concentration of wound odor of a lower level

Examples:

Actisorb Plus	(Johnson & Johnson Medical, Ltd.)
CarboFLEX	ConvaTec, A Bristol-Myers Squibb Company
Carbonet Odor Absorbing Dressing	(Smith & Nephew)
Cliniflex Odour Control Dressing	(CliniMed, Ltd.)
Clinisorb Odour Control Dressing	(CliniMed, Ltd.)
Hollister Odor-Absorbent Dressing	Hollister Incorporated
Kaltocarb	(ConvaTec, Ltd.)
Lyofoam-C	ConvaTec, A Bristol-Myers Squibb Company (Seton Healthcare Group plc)

Collagens

- maintain moist wound environment
- absorb exudate
- conform to wound surface
- enable autolysis of devitalized tissue
- require a secondary dressing

Examples:

ChondroProtec	The Hymed Group
FIBRACOL Collagen-Alginate Wound Dressing	Johnson & Johnson Medical
FIBRACOL Plus Collagen Wound Dressing with Alginate	Johnson & Johnson Medical
hyCOAT	The Hymed Group
hyCURE	Southwest Technologies, Inc.
hyCURE Gel	The Hymed Group
hyCURE Wound Dressing	The Hymed Group
Medifil Gel	BioCore Medical Technologies, Inc.
Medifil Pads	BioCore Medical Technologies, Inc.
Medifil Powder	BioCore Medical Technologies, Inc.
Phyto Derma-Skin Barrier	Aloe Life International
SkinTemp	BioCore Medical Technologies, Inc.

Composites

- nonadherent absorbent pad located in the center
- absorb minimal exudate
- bacteria- and moisture-resistant adhesive dressing

Examples:

3M Microdon Soft Cloth Adhesive Wound Dressing	3M Health Care
Airstrip Island Dressing	Smith & Nephew, Inc. (Smith & Nephew)
Alldress	Mölnlycke
Covaderm Plus V.A.D.	DeRoyal Wound Care
Coverderm Plus	DeRoyal Wound Care

Coverlet Adhesive Dressing	Beiersdorf-Jobst, Inc. (Beiersdorf AG)
Coverlet O.R. Adhesive Surgical Dressing	Beiersdorf-Jobst, Inc. (Beiersdorf AG)
Covertell	Gentell, Inc.
Cutifilm Plus Waterproof Wound Dressing	Beiersdorf-Jobst, Inc. (Beiersdorf AG)
DermaMend Island Dressing	DermaRx Corporation
Melolin	(Smith & Nephew)
MPM Multilayered Dressing	MPM Medical, Inc.
OpSite PLUS	Smith & Nephew, Inc. (Smith & Nephew)
OpSite Post-Op	Smith & Nephew, Inc. (Smith & Nephew)
Soft Wrap	Medline Industries, Inc.
StrataSorb	Medline Industries, Inc.
TELFA PLUS	Kendall Healthcare Products Company
TELFA XTRA	Kendall Healthcare Products Company
VENTEX	Kendall Healthcare Products Company
Viasorb Wound Dressing	Sherwood-Davis & Geck

Contact Layers

- nonadherent
- use on wounds under absorbent cover dressing

Examples:

3M Tegapore Wound Contact Material	3M Health Care
Conformant 2	Smith & Nephew, Inc.

Dermanet	DeRoyal Wound Care
Intersorb Absorbent Gauze Dressings	Sherwood-Davis & Geck
Mepitel	Mölnlycke (SCA Mölnlycke, Ltd.)
N-TERFACE	Winfield Laboratories, Inc.
Owens Dressing	Sherwood-Davis & Geck
Profore Wound Contact Layer	Smith & Nephew, Inc.
Silon-TSR	Bio Med Sciences, Inc.
TELFA Clear	Kendall Healthcare Products Company

Enzymatic Debriding Agents

- destroy necrotic tissue, exudate and/or denatured collagen through proteolytic enzyme action.

Examples:

Accuzyme Papain Urea Debriding Ointment	Healthpoint Medical
Chloresium Ointment	Rystan Company, Inc.
Collagenase SANTYL Ointment	Knoll Pharmaceutical Company
Hurricaine	Beutlich L.P. Pharmaceuticals
Panafil Ointment	Rystan Co., Inc.
Panafil-White Ointment	Rystan Co., Inc.
Phyto Derma-Wound Gel	Aloe Life International

Hydrocolloid Dressings

- contain hydroactive/absorptive particles that interact with wound exudate to form a gelatinous mass
- provide minimal to moderate absorption
- contraindicated when anaerobic infection is suspected

- enable autolysis of devitalized tissue
- may be left on 3 to 7 days
- requires no secondary dressing

Examples: Hydrocolloid wafers

3M Tegasorb Hydrocolloid Dressing	3M Health Care (3M Health Care)
3M Tegasorb THIN Hydrocolloid Dressing	3M Health Care
BGC Matrix	Brennen Medical, Inc.
BioFilm	(Biotrol, Distributed by CliniMed, Ltd.)
CarraSmart Hydrocolloid with Acemannan Hydrogel	Carrington Laboratories, Inc.
COMBI-DERM ACD	ConvaTec, A Bristol-Myers Squibb Company
CombiDerm Non-Adhesive	ConvaTec, A Bristol-Myers Squibb Company
Comfeel Plus Clear Dressing	Coloplast Corporation (Coloplast A/S)
Comfeel Plus Contour Dressing	Coloplast Corporation (Coloplast A/S)
Comfeel Plus Pressure Relief Dressing	Coloplast Corporation (Coloplast A/S)
Comfeel Plus Ulcer Dressing	Coloplast Corporation (Coloplast A/S)
CURADERM Alginate Hydrocolloid Dressing	Kendall Healthcare Products Company
Cutinova hydro	Beiersdorf-Jobst, Inc. (Beiersdorf AG)
Cutinova thin	Beiersdorf-Jobst, Inc. (Beiersdorf AG)
DermaCol Intelligent Hydrocolloid	Derma Sciences, Inc.
DermAssist Hydrocolloid	AssisTec Medical, Inc.

Dermatell Hydrocolloid Wound Dressing	Gentell, Inc.
Dermatell Secure Hydrocolloid Wound Dressing	Gentell, Inc.
DuoDERM CGF BORDER Dressing	ConvaTec, A Bristol-Myers Squibb Company
DuoDERM CGF Control Gel Formula	ConvaTec, A Bristol-Myers Squibb Company
DuoDERM Extra Thin CGF Dressing	ConvaTec, A Bristol-Myers Squibb Company (ConvaTec, Ltd.)
ExuDERM	Medline Industries, Inc.
ExuDERM LP	Medline Industries, Inc.
ExuDERM RCD	Medline Industries, Inc.
Exuderm Sacrum	Medline Industries, Inc.
Exuderm Ultra	Medline Industries, Inc.
Granuflex Bordered	(ConvaTec, Ltd.)
Granuflex Extra Thin	(ConvaTec, Ltd.)
HYDROCOL Hydrocolloid Dressing	Dow Hickam Pharmaceuticals
HYDROCOL Sacral Hydrocolloid Dressing	Dow Hickam Pharmaceuticals
HYDROCOL THIN Hydrocolloid Dressing	Dow Hickam Pharmaceuticals
Hydrocoll	(Hartmann)
RepliCare Hydrocolloid Wound Dressing	Smith & Nephew, Inc.
RepliCare Thin Hydrocolloid Wound Dressing	Smith & Nephew, Inc.
Restore Cx Wound Care Dressing	Hollister Incorporated

Restore Dressing for Psoriasis	Hollister Incorporated
Restore Extra Thin Wound Care Dressing	Hollister Incorporated
Restore Plus Wound Care Dressing	Hollister Incorporated
Restore Wound Care Dressing	Hollister Incorporated
SignaDress Hydrocolloid Dressing	ConvaTec, A Bristol-Myers Squibb Company
Sorbex Hydrocolloid Dressing	Bard Medical Division
Sorbex Thin Hydrocolloid Dressing	Bard Medical Division
SPAND-GEL Sterile Hydrocolloid Occlusive Dressing	Medi-Tech International Corporation
Ultec Hydrocolloid Dressing	Sherwood-Davis & Geck
Ultec Thin Extra Thin Hydrocolloid Dressing	Sherwood-Davis & Geck

Note: Hydrocolloid gels, pastes, and powders may be used in conjunction with hydrocolloid wafers.

Examples: Hydrocolloid gels

Granugel Hydrocolloid Gel	(ConvaTec, Ltd.)

Examples: Hydrocolloid pastes

Comfeel Triad Hydrophilic Wound Dressing	Coloplast Corporation
Comfeel Paste	Coloplast Corporation (Coloplast A/S)
Hydroactive Paste	ConvaTec, A Bristol-Myers Squibb Company
RepliCare Absorbent Paste	Smith & Nephew, Inc.

Examples: Hydrocolloid powders

Comfeel Powder	Coloplast Corporation (Coloplast A/S)
RepliCare Powder	Smith & Nephew, Inc.

Hydrogels

- maintain a clean, moist wound surface
- oxygen-permeable
- cool the surface, can be refrigerated
- absorb minimal exudate
- may require a secondary dressing
- enable autolysis of devitalized tissue

Examples: Amorphous hydrogels

2nd Skin	AFASSCO, Inc.
3M Tegagel Hydrogel Wound Filler	3M Health Care
Bio-Dermal Kit	Kustomer Kinetics Inc.
Biolex Wound Gel	Bard Medical Division
Carrasyn Hydrogel Wound Dressing	Carrington Laboratories Inc.
Carrasyn Spray Gel	Carrington Laboratories Inc.
Carrasyn V (Viscous) Hydrogel Wound Dressing	Carrington Laboratories Inc.
Comfeel Purilon Gel	Coloplast Corporation (Coloplast A/S)
CURAFIL	Kendall Healthcare Products Company
Curasol Gel	Healthpoint Medical
Derma Cool	AFASSCO, Inc.
Dermagran (Zinc Saline) Hydrogel	Derma Sciences, Inc.
Dermagran Hydrophilic B Dressing	Derma Sciences, Inc.
DermaMend Gel	DermaRx Corporation

DiaB Gel Hydrogel Wound Dressing	Carrington Laboratories, Inc.
DuoDERM Hydroactive Gel	ConvaTec, A Bristol-Myers Squibb Company
Elta Dermal Wound Gel	Swiss-American Products, Inc.
Hydrogel Appligard	Gentell, Inc.
Hydrogel Spray Gel	Gentell, Inc.
Hypergel	Mölnlycke
Hyperion Hydrophilic Gel	Hyperion Medical, Inc.
Iamin Gel	Bard Medical Division
IntraSite Gel Hydrogel Wound Dressing	Smith & Nephew, Inc. (Smith & Nephew)
MPM Hydrogel Dressing	MPM Medical, Inc.
Normlgel	Mölnlycke
NU-GEL Collagen Wound Gel	Johnson & Johnson Medical
PanoPlex Hydrogel Wound Dressing	Sage Laboratories, Inc.
Phyto Derma-Wound Gel	Aloe Life International
RadiaCare Gel Hydrogel Wound Dressing	Carrington Laboratories, Inc.
Restore Hydrogel	Hollister Incorporated
SAF-Gel	ConvaTec, A Bristol-Myers Squibb Company
SkinTegrity	Medline Industries, Inc.
SoloSite Wound Gel	Smith & Nephew, Inc.
SPAND-GEL Sterile Hydrogel Amorphous Wound Absorption Dressing Filler	Medi-Tech International Corporation
SteriCare Pre-filled Glycerin Hydrogel Syringes	AssisTec Medical, Inc.
Woun'Dres Natural Collagen Hydrogel	Coloplast Corporation

Examples: Gauze impregnated hydrogels

Biolex Impregnated Wound Dressing	Bard Medical Division
CaraGauze Pads	Carrington Laboratories Inc.
CarraGauze Strips	Carrington Laboratories Inc.
CURAFIL	Kendall Healthcare Products Company
Curasol Gel	Healthpoint Medical
Dermagran Hydrophilic Wound Dressing	Derma Sciences, Inc.
DermaMend Hydrogel Gauze Dressing	DermaRx Corporation
Elta Dermal Impregnated Hydrogel Gauze Pads	Swiss-American Products, Inc.
Hydrogel Impregnated Gauze	Gentell, Inc.
HyFil	B. Braun Medical Inc.
Hyperion Hydrophilic Gel	Hyperion Medical, Inc.
IntraSite Gel Conformable Gauze	(Smith & Nephew)
MPM GelPad Hydrogel Saturated	MPM Medical, Inc.
PanoGauze Non Woven Hydrogel Dressing	Sage Laboratories, Inc.
Restore Hydrogel Impregnated Strip	Hollister Incorporated
SkinTegrity	Medline Industries, Inc.
SteriCare Glycerin Hydrogel	AssisTec Medical, Inc.

Examples: Hydrogel wafers

2nd Skin	AFASSCO, Inc
AcryDerm Advanced Wound Dressing	AcryMed, Inc.

Aquasorb	DeRoyal Wound Care
Aquasorb Border	DeRoyal Wound Care
Aquasorb Border with Covaderm Tape	DeRoyal Wound Care
CarraDres Clear Hydrogel Sheet	Carrington Laboratories Inc.
Carra-Sorb M Freeze-Dried Gel Wound Dressing	Carrington Laboratories Inc.
ClearSite Absorbent Foam Bordered Dressing	ConMed Corporation
ClearSite Absorbent Island Dressing	ConMed Corporation
ClearSite Bandage Roll Dressings	ConMed Corporation
ClearSite Borderless Dressings	ConMed Corporation
CURAGEL	Kendall Healthcare Products Company
Derma Cool	AFASSCO, Inc.
Derma-Gel	Medline Industries, Inc.
DermaMend Hydrogel Sheet	DermaRx Corporation
Elasto-Gel	Southwest Technologies, Inc.
FLEXDERM	Dow Hickam Pharmaceuticals
FlexiGel Sheet	Smith & Nephew, Inc.
Geliperm Sheet	(Geistlich Sons, Ltd.)
NU-GEL Wound Dressing	Johnson & Johnson Medical
RadiaCare Gel Sheet (Clear Hydrogel Sheet)	Carrington Laboratories, Inc.
Spenco 2nd Skin	(Spenco Medical, Ltd.)
THINSite	B. Braun Medical Inc.
Transorbent	B. Braun Medical Inc.

| Vigilon Primary Dressing | Bard Medical Division (Seton Healthcare Group plc) |

Impregnated Gauzes

- nonadherent fine- or open-mesh gauze
- some may enable autolysis of devitalized tissue

Examples:

Aquaphor	Beiersdorf-Jobst, Inc. (Beiersdorf AG)
Clorhexitulle	(Hoechst Marion Roussell, Ltd.)
CURASALT	Kendall Healthcare Products Company
CURITY	Kendall Healthcare Products Company
Dermagran Zinc Saline Dressing	Derma Sciences, Inc.
DermAssist Petrolatum	AssisTec Medical, Inc.
DermAssist Xeroform	AssisTec Medical, Inc.
Fucidin Intertulle	(Leo Laboratories, Ltd.)
Jelonet Paraffin Gauze Dressing	(Smith & Nephew)
Jelonet Petroleum Jelly Gauze Dressing	(Smith & Nephew)
KERLIX	Kendall Healthcare Products Company
Mesalt	Mölnlycke
MPM Gauze Impregnated Saline	MPM Medical, Inc.
Paratulle	(Seton Healthcare Group plc)
Primer Unna Boot	Glenwood
Scarlet Red	Sherwood-Davis & Geck
Serotulle	(Leo Laboratories, Ltd.)

Sofra-Tulle	(Hoechst Marion Roussell, Ltd.)
SPAND-GEL Sterile Impregnated Gauze	Medi-Tech International Corp.
SPAND-GEL Sterile Saline Wet Dressing	Medi-Tech International Corp.
SPAND-GEL Sterile Hydrophor Gauze	Medi-Tech International Corp.
Unitulle	(Hoechst Marion Roussell, Ltd.)
Unna Boot	Tetra Medical Supply Corp.
Vaseline Oil Emulsion Dressing	Sherwood-Davis & Geck
Vaseline Petrolatum Gauze	Sherwood-Davis & Geck
Viscopaste PBT (zinc paste bandage)	Smith & Nephew, Inc.
Xeroflo Gauze Dressing	Sherwood-Davis & Geck
XEROFORM	Kendall Healthcare Products Company
Xeroform Petrolatum Gauze	Sherwood-Davis & Geck

Lubricating Sprays

- provide a protective dressing
- add moisture to epidermis

Examples:

DERMAGRAN Spray	Derma Sciences, Inc.
GRANULEX	Dow Hickam Pharmaceuticals

Moisturizers

- add moisture to epidermis
- assist in maintenance of intact skin

Examples:

3M A & D Emollient Cream	3M Health Care

3M Cavilon Professional Hand Cream	3M Health Care
3M Foot Emollient Cream	3M Health Care
3M One-Step Skin Care Lotion	3M Health Care
After Glove	Kustomer Kinetics, Inc.
Aloe ADE	Kustomer Kinetics, Inc.
Aloe Vesta Skin Cream	ConvaTec, A Bristol-Myers Squibb Company
Antiseptic Skin Cream	Arjo, Inc.
Attrac-Tain Cream	Coloplast Corporation
Body Oils by Skin Savvy	Strong Skin Savvy, Inc.
CV Skin Care Lotion	ConvaTec, A Bristol-Myers Squibb Company
Care-Creme Antimicrobial Cream	Care-Tech Laboratories, Inc.
Carra Derm Moisturizing Cream	Carrington Laboratories, Inc.
Carrington Skin Balm	Carrington Laboratories, Inc.
CURITY	Kendall Healthcare Products Company
DermaMend Barrier	DermaRx Corporation
DiaB Cream	Carrington Laboratories, Inc.
DiaB Daily Care Gel	Carrington Laboratories, Inc.
Elta Creme, The Melting Moisturizer	Swiss-American Products, Inc.
Elta Lite Lotion	Swiss-American Products, Inc.
Elta Lite Tar Lotion	Swiss-American Products, Inc.
Elta Tar Creme	Swiss-American Products, Inc.
Genesis Ointment	Hyperion Medical, Inc.
DermaMend Skin Tear Therapy	DermaRx Corporation

Hand & Skin Lotion	AFASSCO, Inc.
Hand and Body Lotion	Arjo, Inc.
Lantiseptic Therapeutic Cream	Lantiseptic Division, Summit Industries, Inc.
Lotion Soft Body Cream FF	ConvaTec, A Bristol-Myers Squibb Company
Lip Savvy	Strong Skin Savvy, Inc.
Loving Lotion - Topical Antimicrobial	Care-Tech Laboratories, Inc.
MediSkin Extra Care Hand Cream	MediSkin Technology, Inc.
MediSkin Skin Softening Body Lotion	MediSkin Technology, Inc.
MediSkin Skin Soothing Skin Cream	MediSkin Technology, Inc.
MoistureCare Therapeutic Skin Cream	Sage Laboratories, Inc.
Natural Care Gel	Bard Medical Division
Nursing Care Moisturizing Cream	Smith & Nephew, Inc.
Nursing Care Moisturizing Lotion	Smith & Nephew, Inc.
Phyto Derma-Skin Barrier	Aloe Life International
PREVACARE Moisturizing Cream	Johnson & Johnson Medical
PROSHIELD Protective Hand Cream	Healthpoint Medical
PROVON Brand Moisturizing Hand & Body Lotion	PROVON Medical Group
PROVON Brand Perineal Cream	PROVON Medical Group
PROVON Skin Moisturizer with Aloe & Vitamins	PROVON Medical Group

RadiaCare Post Healing Cream	Carrington Laboratories, Inc.
Restore Clean 'N Moist	Hollister Incorporated
Selan Protective Cream and Lotion	P.J. Noyes Company, Inc.
Shield & Protect	Gentell, Inc.
Skin Conditioning Creme	Hollister Incorporated
Skin Magic Antimicrobial Moisturizer	Care-Tech Laboratories, Inc.
Skin Savvy Cream	Strong Skin Savvy, Inc.
Skin Savvy Mist	Strong Skin Savvy, Inc.
Soft Skin After Bath Care	Care-Tech Laboratories, Inc.
Sooth & Cool Inzo	Medline Industries, Inc.
Special Care Cream	Bard Medical Division
Sween Cream	Coloplast Corporation
Swirlsoft Hydrotherapy Dermal Moisturizer	Care-Tech Laboratories, Inc.
TheraSkin Protectant Cream	DeRoyal Wound Care
Third-Step Gel	Bio-Concepts, Inc.
UniCare Moisturizing Lotion	Smith & Nephew, Inc.
UniDerm Moisturizing Cream	Smith & Nephew, Inc.
Vaseline Constant Care Conditioning Cream	Sherwood-Davis & Geck
Xtra-Care Moisturizing Body Lotion	Coloplast Corporation

Nonadherent Dressings

- low adherent, rather than nonadherent
- use on dry or lightly exudating wounds
- can be used as secondary dressing

Examples:

ADAPTIC Non-Adhering Dressing	Johnson & Johnson Medical
Coverlet O.R. Surgical Dressing	DeRoyal Wound Care
CURAD Surgical Adhesive Dressing	Kendall Healthcare Products Company
Cutiplast Wound Dressing	Beiersdorf-Jobst, Inc. (Beiersdorf AG)
DermAssist Oil Emulsion	AssisTec Medical, Inc.
Gauze Pads Non-Adherent	AFASSCO, Inc.
Medline	Medline Industries, Inc.
Melolite Non-adherent Dressing	(Smith & Nephew)
N-A Dressing	(Johnson & Johnson Medical, Ltd.)
N-A Ultra	(Johnson & Johnson Medical, Ltd.)
RELEASE Non-Adhering Dressing	Johnson & Johnson Medical (Johnson & Johnson Medical, Ltd.)
STERI-PAD Gauze Pad	Johnson & Johnson Medical
TELFA	Kendall Healthcare Products (The Kendall Company, Ltd.)
Tricotex	(Smith & Nephew)

Ointments

- provide a petrolatum-based barrier or water-resistant cream against body secretions or chemical injury

Examples:

3M A & D Barrier Ointment	3M Health Care
3M Cavilon Durable Barrier Cream	3M Health Care

3M Zinc Oxide Vanishing Cream	3M Health Care
Aloe Vesta Protective Ointment	ConvaTec, A Bristol-Myers Squibb Company
Barri-Care Antimicrobial Moisture Barrier Ointment	Care-Tech Laboratories, Inc.
BAZA Pro Cream Occlusive Skin Protectant	Coloplast Corporation
Calmoseptine Ointment	Calmoseptine, Inc.
Carrington Moisture Barrier Cream	Carrington Laboratories, Inc.
Carrington Moisture Barrier with Zinc	Carrington Laboratories, Inc.
Dermagran Ointment	Derma Sciences, Inc.
Double Guard Skin Protectant	Bard Medical Division
Dyprotex Rash Ointment Pads	Blistex, Inc.
ELTA Seal Moisture Barrier	Swiss-American Products, Inc.
iLEX Skin Protectant Paste	ConvaTec, A Bristol-Myers Squibb Company
INZO	Medline Industries, Inc.
Lantiseptic Skin Protectant	Lantiseptic Division, Summit Industries, Inc.
Moisture Barrier Ointment	Mentor - Health Care Products
Nursing Care Protective Ointment	Smith & Nephew, Inc.
Peri-Care Moisture Barrier Ointment	Coloplast Corporation
PREVACARE Extra Protective Ointment	Johnson & Johnson Medical
PREVACARE Personal Protective Cream	Johnson & Johnson Medical

PROSHIELD PLUS Skin Protectant	Healthpoint Medical
PROVON Brand Moisturizing Perineal Barrier	PROVON Medical Group
PROVON Brand Perineal Barrier	PROVON Medical Group
Restore Barrier Creme Skin Protectant	Hollister Incorporated
Restore Clean 'N Moist Skin Protectant	Hollister Incorporated
Selan + Zinc Oxide Barrier Cream	P.J. Noyes Company, Inc.
Shield & Protect Moisture/Barrier Cream	Gentell, Inc.
Soothe & Cool Moisture Barrier Ointment	Medline Industries, Inc.
Special Care Moisture Barrier Ointment	Bard Medical Division
TheraSkin Barrier Ointment	DeRoyal Wound Care
Triple Care Protective Cream	Smith & Nephew, Inc.
Triple Care EPC Extra Protective Cream	Smith & Nephew, Inc.
Uni Salve Protective Ointment	Smith & Nephew, Inc.
Vaseline Constant Care Moisture Barrier Salve	Sherwood-Davis & Geck
Vaseline Petroleum Jelly	Sherwood-Davis & Geck

Semipermeable Foam Dressings

- absorb exudate while maintaining a moist wound surface
- have a hydrophobic outer surface
- enable autolysis of devitalized tissue

Examples:

3M Reston Self-Adhering Foam Products	3M Health Care
Adhesive Cloth Dressings	Ferris Manufacturing Corporation
Adhesive Urethane Dressings	Ferris Manufacturing Corporation
Allevyn Adhesive Dressing	Smith & Nephew, Inc. (Smith & Nephew)
Allevyn Cavity Wound Dressing	Smith & Nephew, Inc. (Smith & Nephew)
Allevyn Hydrophilic Polyurethane Foam Dressing	Smith & Nephew, Inc. (Smith & Nephew)
Allevyn Tracheostomy	Smith & Nephew, Inc. (Smith & Nephew)
BIOPATCH Antimicrobial Dressing	Johnson & Johnson Medical
CarraSmart Foam Dressing	Carrington Laboratories, Inc.
CURAFOAM	Kendall Healthcare Products Company
Cutinova foam	Beiersdorf-Jobst, Inc. (Beiersdorf AG)
DermaMend Cavity Filler	DermaRx Corporation
DermaMend Foam	DermaRx Corporation
Epigard	Ormed
Epitech	Rynel, Ltd.
Flexipore FLEXZAN	(Polymedica) Dow Hickam Pharmaceuticals
Hydrasorb	ConvaTec, A Bristol-Myers Squibb Company
Lo Profile Foam	Gentell, Inc.

Lyofoam	ConvaTec, A Bristol-Myers Squibb Company (Seton Healthcare Group plc)
Lyofoam A	ConvaTec, A Bristol-Myers Squibb Company
Lyofoam C	ConvaTec, A Bristol-Myers Squibb Company
Lyofoam Extra	ConvaTec, A Bristol-Myers Squibb Company (Seton Healthcare Group plc)
Lyofoam T	ConvaTec, A Bristol-Myers Squibb Company
Non-Adhesive Membrane Pad Dressings	Ferris Manufacturing Corporation
Non-Adhesive Membrane Roll Dressings	Ferris Manufacturing Corporation
NU-DERM Foam Island Dressing	Johnson & Johnson Medical
Polyderm Border with Convaderm Tape	DeRoyal Wound Care
PolyTube Tube-Site Dressing	Ferris Manufacturing Corporation
SPAND-GEL Sterile Foam Dressing	Medi-Tech International Corporation
Spyroflex	(BritCair)
Spyrosorb (Adhesive)	(BritCair)
TIELLE Hydropolymer Dressing	Johnson & Johnson Medical (Johnson & Johnson Medical, Ltd.)
VigiFOAM Dressing	Bard Medical Division

Skin Sealants

- provide protection from mechanical and chemical injury
- provide a copolymer film on skin
- most contain alcohol

Examples:

3M No Sting Barrier Film	3M Health Care
Allkare Protective Barrier Wipe	ConvaTec, A Bristol-Myers Squibb Company
Bard Incontinence Barrier Film	Bard Medical Division
Bard Protective Barrier Film	Bard Medical Division
Hollister Skin Gel	Hollister Incorporated
Hollister Skin Gel Protective Dressing Wipe	Hollister Incorporated
No-Sting Skin-Prep	Smith & Nephew, Inc.
Prep-Site	Acme United Corporation
PREPPIES Skin Barrier Wipe	Kendall Healthcare Products Company
Shield Skin Protective Barrier	Mentor - Health Care Products
Skin-Prep Protective Dressing	Smith & Nephew, Inc.
Sureprep	Medline Industries, Inc.
Sween Prep Protective Skin Barrier	Coloplast Corporation
Sween Prep	Coloplast Corporation

Specialty Absorptive Dressings

- are low adherent
- are for use on dry or lightly exudating wounds
- can be used as secondary dressings

Examples:

3M Tegaderm Transparent Dressing w/Absorbent Pad	3M Health Care
BreakAway	Winfield Laboratories, Inc.
Breast Vest	Smith & Nephew, Inc.

Chest Vest	Smith & Nephew, Inc.
Clearsite Hydrogauze Dressings	ConMed Corporation
Covaderm	DeRoyal Wound Care
Epigard	Ormed
Exu-Dry Wound Dressing	Smith & Nephew, Inc.
Intersorb Absorbent Gauze Dressings	Sherwood-Davis & Geck
Iodoflex Pad	Healthpoint Medical
Iodosorb Gel	Healthpoint Medical
Mepore	Mölnlycke (SCA Mölnlycke, Ltd.)
Multipad	DeRoyal Wound Care
Primapore Adhesive Wound Dressing	Smith & Nephew, Inc. (Smith & Nephew)
Sofsorb	DeRoyal Wound Care
TIELLE Hydropolymer Dressing	Johnson & Johnson Medical

Transparent Adhesive Dressings

- are semipermeable, sterile, and waterproof
- create a moist environment
- are nonabsorptive
- enable autolysis of devitalized tissue
- create a "second skin" and protect against friction

Examples:

3M Tegaderm HP Transparent Dressing	3M Health Care
3M Tegaderm Transparent Dressing	3M Health Care (3M Health Care)
ACU-derm	Acme United Corporation
Advanced Film	Hyperion Medical, Inc.
Arglaes (antimicrobial)	Medline Industries, Inc.

BIOCLUSIVE MVP Select Transparent Dressing	Johnson & Johnson Medical
BIOCLUSIVE Select Transparent Dressing	Johnson & Johnson Medical
BIOCLUSIVE Transparent Dressing	Johnson & Johnson Medical (Johnson & Johnson Medical, Ltd.)
BlisterFilm Transparent Dressing	Sherwood-Davis & Geck
CarraFilm Transparent Film Dressing	Carrington Laboratories Inc.
CarraSmart Film (High MVTR) Transparent Film Dressing	Carrington Laboratories Inc.
DEKNAFLEX	(Smith & Nephew)
DermaFilm Intelligent Film Dressing	Derma Sciences, Inc.
DermaSite Transparent Film Dressing	Derma Sciences, Inc.
DermAssist Transparent Film	AssisTec Medical, Inc.
EpiVIEW	ConvaTec, A Bristol-Myers Squibb Company
FLEXFILM	Dow Hickam Pharmaceuticals
Opraflex	Professional Medical Products, Inc.
OpSite	Smith & Nephew, Inc.
OpSite Flexifix	Smith & Nephew, Inc. (Smith & Nephew)
OpSite FLEXIGRID	Smith & Nephew, Inc. (Smith & Nephew)
OpSite IV3000	Smith & Nephew, Inc. (Smith & Nephew)
POLYSKIN II	Kendall Healthcare Products Company

POLYSKIN MR	Kendall Healthcare Products Company
ProCyte Transparent Film Dressing	Bard Medical Division
Reactic	(Smith & Nephew)
Suresite	Medline Industries, Inc.
Transeal	DeRoyal Wound Care
UniFlex Transparent Dressing	Smith & Nephew, Inc.

Wound Cleansers

- apply directly into wound for cleaning
- use 35-ml syringe with 19-gauge needle or angiocath
- clean wound at every dressing change
- see package insert for indications and contra-indications

Types of wound cleansers include:

- **Acetic acid**
  Appropriate for *Pseudomonas*; toxic to fibroblasts.
- **Potassium hypochlorite**
  Appropriate for *Staphlococcus* and *Streptococcus*; toxic to fibroblasts.
- **Hydrogen peroxide**
  Provides mechanical debridement; toxic to fibroblasts.
- **Normal saline**
  Always appropriate for granulating wounds.
- **Povidone-iodine**
  Broad-spectrum antimicrobial; toxic to fibroblasts.

Examples:

Allclenz Wound Cleanser	Healthpoint Medical
Biolex Wound Cleanser	Bard Medical Division
Brennen Sterile Saline Solution Spray	Brennen Medical Inc.
Burn Septic	AFASSCO, Inc.

Carra-Klenz Wound & Skin Cleanser	Carrington Laboratories Inc.
Chloresium Solution	Rystan Co., Inc.
Clinical Care Wound Cleanser	Care-Tech Laboratories, Inc.
Clinswound	Sage Laboratories, Inc.
Comfeel Sea-Clens	Coloplast Corporation
Constant Clens Dermal Wound Cleanser	Sherwood-Davis & Geck
CURAKLENSE	Kendall Healthcare Products Company
DEBRISAN Wound Cleaning Beads	Johnson & Johnson Medical (Pharmacia, Ltd.) (Upjohn, Ltd.)
DEBRISAN Wound Cleaning Paste	Johnson & Johnson Medical (Pharmacia, Ltd.) (Upjohn, Ltd.)
Dermagran Wound Cleanser with Zinc	Derma Sciences, Inc.
Dermal Wound Cleanser	Smith & Nephew, Inc.
DermaMend Antimicrobial Cleanser	DermaRx Corporation
DiaB Klenz Wound Cleanser	Carrington Laboratories Inc.
Elta Dermal Wound Cleanser	Swiss-American Products, Inc.
Genesis Cleansers	Hyperion Medical, Inc.
Gentell Wound Cleanser	Gentell, Inc.
hyCARE	The Hymed Group
Hygenique Plus	Andermac, Inc
Iamin Wound Cleanser	Bard Medical Division
Lobana Saline Wound Cleanser	Lobana Laboratories
Medi Wipes	AFASSCO, Inc.

131

Micro-Klenz Antiseptic Wound Cleanser	Carrington Laboratories Inc.
MPM Anti-Microbial Wound Cleanser	MPM Medical, Inc.
MPM Wound & Skin Cleanser	MPM Medical, Inc.
Proshield Foam and Spray	Healthpoint Medical
Proshield Kit	Healthpoint Medical
Proshield Spray	Healthpoint Medical
Puri-Clens Wound Deodorizer, Spray Gel	Coloplast Corporation
RadiaCare Klenz Wound Cleanser	Carrington Laboratories Inc.
Restore Wound Cleanser	Hollister, Incorporated
SAF-Clens Chronic Wound Cleanser	ConvaTec, A Bristol-Myers Squibb Company
SeptiCare Antimicrobial Wound Cleanser	Sage Laboratories, Inc.
Shur-Clens Wound Cleanser	ConvaTec, A Bristol-Myers Squibb Company
SPAND-GEL Wound Cleanser	Medi-Tech International Corporation
Techni-Care – Microbicide	Care-Tech Laboratories Inc.
Ultra-Klenz Wound & Skin Cleanser	Carrington Laboratories Inc.
Wound Cleanser	Gentell, Inc.

Wound Fillers

- absorb exudate
- fill dead space
- conform to wound surface
- keep the wound surface clean and moist
- enable autolysis of devitalized tissue

Examples:

AcryDerm STRANDS Absorbent Wound Dressing	AcryMed, Inc.
Bard Absorption Dressing	Bard Medical Division
Biafine RE	KCI
Biafine WDE	KCI
CAVI-CARE	(Smith & Nephew)
Chronicure (wound exudate absorber)	Derma Sciences, Inc.
Cutinova cavity	Beiersdorf-Jobst, Inc. (Beiersdorf AG)
Debrisan Absorbent Pad	(Pharmacia, Ltd.) (Upjohn, Ltd.)
hyCURE	Southwest Technologies, Inc.
HydraGran Absorbent Dressing	Allegiance Healthcare Corporation
MPM Hydrogel Dressing	MPM Medical, Inc.
Multidex	DeRoyal Wound Care
OsmoCyte PCA Pillow Dressing	Bard Medical Division
OsmoCyte Pillow Dressing	Bard Medical Division
Polywic Wound Filler	Ferris Manufacturing Corporation
SteriCare Copolymer Absorbent Powder	AssisTec Medical, Inc.

Wound Pouches

- look like ostomy pouches with or without attached skin barrier
- can be cut to fit wound shape and size
- some have hinged caps that allow for treatment or inspection
- can be adapted for continuous drainage

Examples:

Bongort Max-E-Pouch	Smith & Nephew, Inc.
Wound Drainage Collector	Hollister Incorporated
Wound Manager	ConvaTec, A Bristol-Myers Squibb Company

Miscellaneous Wound Care Products

- see package insert for instructions on usage
- may require physician order

Examples: Biosynthetics

BIOBRANE	Dow Hickam Pharmaceuticals
E-Z Derm	Brennen Medical, Inc.
Humatrix Microclysmic Gel	Care-Tech Laboratories, Inc.
Inerpan Wound Dressings	Sherwood-Davis & Geck
Mediskin	Brennen Medical, Inc.

Examples: Growth factors

REGRANEX (becaplermin) Gel 0.01%	Ortho-McNeil Pharmaceutical

Examples: Hydrofibers

AQUACEL HYDROFIBER Wound Dressing	ConvaTec, A Bristol-Myers Squibb Company (ConvaTec, Ltd.)

BIBLIOGRAPHY

Alguire PC, Mathes BM. Chronic venous insufficiency and venous ulceration. J Gen Intern Med 1997;12:374-83.

American Diabetes Association. Foot care in patients with diabetes mellitus. Diabetes Care 1998;21:S54-S55.

Apelqvist J. Wound healing in diabetes: outcome and costs. Clin Podiatr Med Surg 1998;15:21-39.

Armstrong DG, Lavery LA, Wunderlich RP. Risk factors for diabetic foot ulceration: a logical approach to treatment. J Wound Ostomy Continence Nurs 1998;25:123-8.

Bergstrom N, et al. Treatment of pressure ulcers. Clinical Practice Guideline, No. 15. AHCPR Publication No. 95-0652. Rockville, MD: Agency for Health Care Policy and Research, Public Health Service, U.S. Department of Health and Human Services; 1994.

Castronuovo JJ, Adera HM, Smiell JM, Price RM. Skin perfusion measurement is valuable in the diagnosis of critical limb ischemia. J Vasc Surg 1997;26:629-37.

Criado E, Farber MA, Marston WA, Daniel PF, Burnham CB, Keagy BA. The role of air plethysmography in the diagnosis of chronic venous insufficiency. J Vasc Surg 1998;27:660-70.

Eaglstein WH, Falanga V. Tissue engineering and the development of Apligraf®, a human skin equivalent. Clin Ther 1997;19:894-905.

Edelson GW. Systemic and nutritional considerations in diabetic wound healing. Clin Podiatr Med Surg 1998;15:41-8.

Falanga V, Eaglstein WH. Leg and foot ulcers: a clinician's guide. London: Martin Dunitz Limited; 1995.

Fantl JA, et al. Urinary incontinence in adults: acute and chronic management. Clinical Practice Guideline, Number 2, 1996 Update. AHCPR Publication No. 96-0682. Rockville, MD: Agency for Health Care Policy and Research, Public Health Service, U.S. Department of Health and Human Services; 1996.

Gogia P. Clinical wound management. Thorofare, New Jersey: Slack, Inc.; 1995.

Goode PS, Thomas DR. Pressure ulcers: local wound care. Clin Geriatr Med 1997;13:543-52.

Henderson CT, Ayello EA, Sussman C, Leiby DM, Bennett MA,

Dungog EF, Sprigle S, Woodruff L. Draft definition of Stage I pressure ulcers: inclusion of persons with darkly pigmented skin. Adv Wound Care 1997;10(5):16-9.

Hess CT. Nurse's clinical guide to wound care, 2nd ed. Springhouse, PA: Springhouse Corporation; 1998.

Jeter KF, Lutz JB. Skin care in the frail, elderly, dependent, incontinent patient. Adv Wound Care 1996;9(1):29-34.

Johannsen F, Gam AN, Karlsmark T. Ultrasound therapy in chronic leg ulceration: a meta-analysis. Wound Rep Reg 1998;6:121-6.

Kozak GP, Campbell DR, Frykberg RG, Habershaw GM, editors. Management of diabetic foot problems, 2nd ed. Philadelphia: W.B. Saunders Company; 1995.

Maklebust J. Pressure ulcer assessment. Clin Geriatr Med 1997;13:455-81.

Maklebust J, Sieggreen M. Pressure ulcers: guidelines for prevention and nursing management, 2nd ed. Springhouse, PA: Springhouse Corporation; 1996.

McLeod AG. Principles of alternating pressure surfaces. Adv Wound Care 1997;10(7):30-6.

Morison M, Moffatt C. A colour guide to the assessment and management of leg ulcers, 2nd ed. London: Times Mirror International Publishers Limited; 1994.

Panel for the Prediction and Prevention of Pressure Ulcers in Adults. Pressure ulcers in adults: prediction and prevention. Clinical Practice Guideline, No. 3. AHCPR Publication No. 92-0047. Rockville, MD: Agency for Health Care Policy and Research, Public Health Service, U.S. Department of Health and Human Services; 1992.

Rockson SG, Cooke JP. Peripheral arterial insufficiency: mechanisms, natural history, and therapeutic options. Adv Intern Med 1998;43:253-77.

Rubano JJ, Kerstein MD. Arterial insufficiency and vasculitides. J Wound Ostomy Continence Nurs 1998;25:147-57.

Suh DY, Hunt TK. Time line of wound healing. Clin Podiatr Med Surg 1998;15:1-9.

Sussman C, Bates-Jensen B, editors. Wound care: a collaborative practice manual for physical therapists and nurses. Gaithersburg, MD: Aspen Publishers, Inc.; 1998.

Thomas DR. Specific nutritional factors in wound healing. Adv Wound Care 1997;10(4):40-3.

Wysocki AB. A review of the skin and its appendages. Adv Wound Care 1995;8(2):53-70; see erratum, 1995;8(4):8.